Natural Cures for the Common Cold

Natural Cures for the Common Cold

Powerful, Drug-Free Remedies
Proven to Work

Carol Turkington

HARBOR PRESS

GIG HARBOR, WASHINGTON

Library of Congress Cataloging-in-Publication Data

Turkington, Carol.
    Natural cures for the common cold : powerful, drug-free remedies
proven to work / Carol Turkington.
        p.   cm.
    Includes bibliographical references and index.
    ISBN 0-936197-38-2
        1. Cold (Disease) — Treatment.   2. Cold (Disease) — Popular works.
3. Naturopathy.   I. Title.
RF361.T87 1999   98-35534
616.2'05 — dc21   CIP

ISBN: 0-936197-38-2

IMPORTANT NOTICE:

NATURAL CURES FOR THE COMMON COLD
Powerful, Drug-Free Remedies Proven to Work

Printed in the United States of America
1 3 5 7 9 10 8 6 4 2

Harbor Press, Inc.
P.O. Box 1656
Gig Harbor, WA 98335

Contents

Foreword

 AVING A COLD is a very humbling experience in today's fast-paced world. We're used to drive-through food, drive-through money machines, and drive-through drugstores. We drink instant coffee, have day surgery, and use cell phones and fax machines. But what happens when we have a cold? We can't seem to find that quick, simple solution. Symptoms last seven days when we take drugs, and a week when we don't.

Natural Cures for the Common Cold offers you an alternative to the myriad of ineffective, expensive cold medications that most of us take almost automatically at the first sign of a cold. Not only do these medications not work most of the time, many have unpleasant and sometimes harmful side effects. In this book, you'll find a wide range of simple, drug-free treatments for every symptom of the common cold. Whether you're battling a fever, sore throat, cough, nausea, or just general aches and pains, you'll find a safe, natural remedy that works for you.

Carol Turkington has selected the best natural home remedies available from scores of well-respected physicians and other health professionals, and she has presented them in a way that will make it easy for you to choose those that best meet your particular needs. From herbal teas and soups, to "healing foods" like mushrooms and chicken soup, to simple self-massage techniques, there's something here for everyone.

Enjoy this unique guide and use it as soon as you feel a cold coming on. Relax, read a good book, sip comforting teas, excuse yourself from all but the most necessary activities, and experiment with the natural treatments that follow. You'll find simple, inexpensive, nontoxic home remedies that will get you back on your feet quickly— and help you keep your immune system strong enough to fight off the next cold.

Michele Moore, M.D.
Keene, New Hampshire

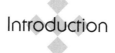

Introduction

ACH WEEK IN WINTER, 26 million Americans come down
with some version of the common cold—an illness that
has been the bane of doctors since the first physician applied the first leech in a vain attempt to ease the sniffles.
Hippocrates thought that colds were caused by too much "waste
matter" in the brain. A runny nose, he reasoned, was simply the
brain's way of cleaning house. In Rome, cold sufferers were advised
to kiss the furry snout of a mouse. But it wasn't until the great 12th
century physician Moses Maimonides came up with his chicken soup
remedy that physicians had any real weapon to use against cold symptoms at all. Unhappily, scientists since then have made precious little
headway in finding an effective method to cure the common cold.
Not for lack of trying, however—store shelves are lined with hundreds of expensive, multi-symptom cold medicines that at best don't
work and at worst, can lead to a range of harmful side effects.

The fact that most of these expensive cold remedies don't work
shouldn't really be surprising, since the cold may be described as
"common," but it's actually quite complex. Colds are caused not by
one type of virus, but by *200 different viruses* of various sizes and

shapes, each one capable of causing a different version of the common cold.

Clearly, the common cold shows no signs of going away. And because most conventional treatments just don't work, millions of sufferers are turning to natural solutions such as herbs, special diets, acupuncture, massage, visualization, and others in an attempt to find a cure.

In this easy-to-use guide, you'll find dozens of effective all-natural ways to treat each and every symptom of the common cold, from headaches to upset stomachs. These treatments, which can all be carried out in your own home, don't involve drugs or prescription medicines. They are simple natural remedies used or advocated by doctors and other health professionals around the world. Some are thousands of years old, yet still the most powerful cures for your cold symptoms.

This book provides you with drug-free, noninvasive, inexpensive, and effective ways to:

- relieve a sore throat
- cope with chills
- reduce fever
- ease aches and pains
- stop headaches
- clear congested sinuses and a runny nose
- soothe an upset stomach
- arrest a cough

Moreover, you'll learn why over-the-counter medications don't work for most symptoms of the common cold. Lists of specific products under each drug class are provided to help you identify individual drugs and the symptoms they're supposed to treat. You'll also find a section devoted to preventing the common cold both at home and at work. In addition, each section of the book includes recipes for brews, soups, and other foods that are designed to ease specific complaints.

While most of the symptoms of a cold are more irritating than life-threatening, there are times when certain symptoms demand medical attention. Each section will include warning boxes, where appropriate, to help you decide when your symptoms may indicate a more serious problem—and what to do about it.

CHAPTER ONE

Why Over-the-Counter Cold Medications Don't Work

L ET'S FACE IT. Modern medicine just hasn't found any medication that works against the more than 200 viruses that cause the common cold. When researchers reviewed 51 studies of nonprescription cold formulas published from 1950 to 1991, they found that cold remedies don't affect a cold's severity or duration since they do nothing to attack cold viruses or boost the immune system's fight against them. At best, all you can expect from a cold preparation is the suppression of symptoms: modest relief from nasal congestion, runny nose, or cough. At worst, there are often uncomfortable and sometimes harmful side effects. And keep in mind that research has found that most of these products don't work at all on children under age five. But when you're sick, you want relief—so you usually go to the local drug store, where you try to choose a cold remedy from the more than 2,800 products on the shelves. According to research, the choice of cold medicines is so overwhelming that while most shoppers spend just about five seconds choosing an average drugstore item, they take two and a half minutes to select a cold medication.

Should you pick caplets or gelcaps, capsules or pills? Elixir or cough medicine, multi-symptom relief, cough-and-cold, sinus and allergy relief—or throw in the towel and just grab a box of acetaminophen? With each manufacturer packaging their products in four or five different ways, it's hard to know which to choose. One company's "cough and cold" remedy contains very different medicine from another's "cold and cough" product. And Chlor-Trimeton (the former brand name for the simple antihistamine chlorpheniramine) is now the name for eight different variations, one of which has no antihistamine at all.

The product names can also be confusing. For example, a box labeled "allergy sinus" might have exactly the same ingredients as one called "cold and flu." That's why it's important to study the ingredients listed on the box. Nearly all cold remedies contain some combination of decongestants, antihistamines, pain relievers, and cough suppressants.

Since only a few ingredients are really considered effective against a cold, most of the differences between these products are really just in the flavors or in the delivery system (pill, capsule, caplet, elixir, or gel cap).

Why Multi-symptom Remedies Don't Work

Most people buy multi-symptom remedies when they have a cold. In fact, more than $1 billion a year is spent on all-in-one cold formulas. Yet most doctors discourage patients from taking them. Why?

1. *Multi-symptom medications are expensive and ineffective*, according to Stephen R. Jones, M.D., chief of medicine at Good Samaritan Hospital and Medical Center in Portland, Oregon. They contain ingredients to relieve every major cold symptom, but since these symptoms don't develop all at once, you're paying for medicine you don't need. Since you don't usually get all of the symptoms of a cold at once, why take a medicine that is designed to work against

symptoms you don't have? If you've got a typical upper respiratory cold, you'll probably start out with a sore throat and a feeling of body aches, followed by congestion and then a runny nose. Then you'll start to sneeze and cough. If at the first sign of a sore throat you start taking a multi-symptom pill, you're really taking much more medication than you need at the moment. Why pay for a cough suppressant when what's really bothering you is a stuffy nose? And why risk side effects from medications you may not need?

For example, if you're suffering with lots of head cold symptoms but you're not really coughing, taking a combination product will deliver cough medicine that you don't need and an antihistamine that may put you to sleep. If your cold symptoms are mainly sneezing and coughing, taking a multi-symptom product will deliver unnecessary decongestants which will make you feel jumpy and on edge.

2. *Popular cold remedies may actually inhibit the body's immune responses while they suppress cold symptoms.* Keep in mind that most of your symptoms are not caused by the cold virus. They are triggered by the body's natural response in its battle against the invading microbes. By suppressing these symptoms, you may actually be making your cold last longer. For example, since a mild fever (anything under 102 degrees F) actually boosts your body's ability to fight the cold virus, it's a good idea to try to avoid lowering the fever.

❖❖❖CAUTION: If you're over age 60, you have heart disease, or any immune-impairing illness, contact your doctor at the first sign of fever.

3. *All drugs—even over-the-counter products—carry some risk, especially for people with certain types of medical conditions.* The more ingredients a drug has, the greater the risk of an unpleasant reaction. Moreover, many OTC drugs, when mixed with prescription medicines, can cause serious problems.

For example, if you take a decongestant, which can raise your blood pressure, on top of antidepressants or diet pills, it can send your blood pressure through the roof. Since some over-the-counter cold preparations are designed to be long-acting with various ingredients released at different times, if you do have side effects it may take too much time for your body to eliminate the drug, creating a health risk.

4. *You could inadvertently overmedicate yourself by adding other drugs such as painkillers along with a combination cold product that already contains one.*

5. *Taking a multi-symptom preparation locks you into a set dosage.* This means you can't increase or decrease the dosage of one ingredient as your symptoms change. If you're taking a cold formula preparation and your headache goes away before the rest of your symptoms, you're still taking, for example, 1,000 mg. of acetaminophen every six hours for nothing.

6. *Some all-in-one products contain a combination of ingredients that is just plain illogical.* For example, one cough syrup contains an ingredient that loosens phlegm (making it easier to cough up) while another ingredient in the same product suppresses coughing.

7. *Combination products that pack a variety of medications into one pill are usually more expensive than a generic version of just one individual drug aimed at easing one particular symptom.*

Single-Action Cold Medications: What You Need to Know

The drug-free approach to dealing with the common cold is by far the best path to getting well. But if your symptoms are really troublesome, you may feel that as a last resort you must take an over-the-counter medicine to cope. In this case, most experts recommend single-action remedies as opposed to the multi-symptom medicines that aim for the shotgun approach.

If you want to clear up your nose, for example, pick a decongestant. If your head and body are aching, choose a pain reliever such as ibuprofen or acetaminophen. For a nagging cough, choose a cough suppressant and suck on medicated lozenges, or use a spray to ease your scratchy throat.

Here are descriptions of the most common single-action cold remedies, and why, for the most part, they should be avoided.

ANALGESICS (PAINKILLERS)

aspirin
acetaminophen (Tylenol, Datril)
ibuprofen (Advil, Medipren, Nuprin)
naproxen sodium (Aleve)

The most common analgesics, or painkillers, are acetaminophen, ibuprofen, and aspirin. At the first sign of a sore throat, you can ease the pain by taking one of these three, but only aspirin and ibuprofen will reduce inflammation. Taken for a short time, most experts believe these pain relievers don't pose a risk. However, over-the-counter nonnarcotic analgesics should only be used for 48 hours before seeking medical advice.

One of the problems with taking these drugs is that they may mask a fever, which can be an important clue to the development of further infection. In many cases, it's best to let a mild fever run its course, since a fever is actually a valuable weapon in the anti-cold virus arsenal.

In addition, some studies have found a possible link to liver and kidney damage after long-term use of acetaminophen, or when it is combined with heavy drinking. Aspirin may irritate the stomach lining. Children should avoid aspirin, since it has been linked with Reye's syndrome, a potentially deadly disorder in kids who have flu or chicken pox, both of which initially look a lot like the common cold.

ANESTHETIC AGENTS

Benzocaine

While anesthetic agents such as benzocaine, are useful for the temporary relief of minor sore throat pain, the most common dosage form, lozenges, must be dissolved slowly in the mouth, not bitten or chewed. Because of this, in many cases, the anesthetic never reaches the throat.

ANTIBIOTICS

Antibiotics are very effective against bacteria—*but bacteria don't cause colds. Let's say it again—antibiotics are ineffective against viruses, and viruses cause colds.* Moreover, when you take antibiotics, they will kill the helpful bacteria you have in your body. You can also become allergic to antibiotics by repeatedly using them. Finally, bacteria become resistant to antibiotics after they have been exposed to these drugs often enough. After repeated courses of antibiotics, organisms may successfully change their structure so they will be less affected by the antibiotic the next time. When you are really sick with a bacterial infection and need an antibiotic, that antibiotic may no longer be effective in your body against bacteria causing the illness.

Antibiotics Don't Cure Colds

Antibiotics are prescribed for viral infections all too often in this country when they just aren't effective. This overuse has real repercussions: it's not just a waste of money, but prescribing antibiotics too freely has led to the development of superbacteria that no longer respond to any antibiotic at all.

How to tell if your symptoms are caused by a virus? You most likely have a viral infection (meaning antibiotics won't help) if you have any of the following symptoms for less than one week:

- scratchy throat
- runny nose
- watery eyes
- sneezing
- minor headache
- minor aches and pains
- fatigue

You probably have a bacterial infection if you have any of the following:

- throat that is very sore or inflamed, or that produces pus
- pain or problems swallowing
- swollen glands in your neck
- fever above 100 degrees F
- severe headache for more than 24 hours
- tenderness over sinuses
- persistent extreme listlessness
- persistent coughing, wheezing, breathlessness
- chest pain when coughing or breathing
- yellow, green, brown, or rusty phlegm

ANTIHISTAMINES

Actifed (DM; with Codeine Cough) CoTylenol Cold Medication
brampheniramine (Dimetapp) Dimetapp-DM (and Codeine)
chlorpheniramine maleate (Chlor-Trimeton)
Dramamine diphenhydramine (Benadryl)
Novahistaine Benylin
NyQuil Nighttime Colds Chlor-Amine
PediaCare 3 Children's Cold clemastine fumarate (Tavist)
Pertussin (AM and PM) Co-Actifed Robitussin
Contac Severe Cold Formula Sominex liquid
Triminic Expectorant

All in all, there's just no scientific basis for using antihistamines to treat a common cold, according to Karen Tietze, an associate professor of clinical pharmacy who wrote the chapter on cold medicines in the *Handbook of Nonprescription Drugs*, published by the American Pharmaceutical Association. Studies have found that antihistamines are ineffective against most symptoms of the common cold because colds don't produce histamines, which these drugs are designed to fight. Histamines are produced in allergic reactions, but are NOT triggered by the invasion of common cold viruses.

Antihistamines dry up already-irritated mucous membranes, according to David N. Bilbert, M.D., director of the Department of Medical Education at Providence Medical Center in Portland, Oregon. They thicken the nasal mucus so you feel more like you need more decongestants, and they can cause coughs. In addition to drowsiness, their other side effects are uncomfortable: dry eyes, nose, and mouth, and impaired motor skills. In fact, these medications can make you so sleepy, they are the main ingredients in "P.M." formulas.

In addition, recent research in the *Journal of the National Cancer Institute* suggests that antihistamines might actually spur tumor growth. Apparently, antihistamines share similar chemical structure with the chemical DPPE, used in cancer research to promote tumor growth. When Canadian researchers injected mice with two types of tumor cells and then gave some of them antihistamines, the largest tumors were found in those who had been given the antihistamines.

There is one benefit to antihistamines: they are most useful in treating allergy symptoms such as a runny nose. If your sneezing is driving you crazy, research suggests that antihistamines can reduce sneezing by 50 percent, according to leading cold researcher Jack Gwaltney, M.D., chief of virology at the University of Virginia's medical school. However, even if they're used just to stop sneezing, research suggests that only one antihistamine of the five commonly used (chlorpheniramine) really helps to dry up a runny nose. The differences between antihistamines in the products listed here are primarily in their side effects, the most common of which is drowsiness.

COUGH MEDICINES (ANTITUSSIVES)

EXPECTORANTS: *guainfenesin (Robitussin DM)*

SUPPRESSANTS: *dextromethorphan (Robitussin DM, Robitussin Cough, Calmers)*

When faced with a persistent cough, most people turn to over-the-counter preparations for relief, but natural, home-made cough syrups are just as effective. For recipes on specific natural cough remedies, see Chapter Nine.

Natural remedies work just as well as expensive cough preparations—with no harmful side effects. But if you do use drugs, you need to know that drugs that inhibit your cough are classified into two groups: those that act in the lungs and airways (peripheral drugs) and those that act in the brain (central drugs). Central drugs, such as codeine, are usually most effective, but they have side effects, such as drowsiness and constipation, and codeine can be addictive.

If you're considering an OTC cough medicine, the first thing to ask yourself is, What kind of cough do I have? A dry, hacking cough (what your doctor calls unproductive) will respond best to a central drug formula with codeine (available without prescription in some states) or dextromethorphan. These medications, which are also called antitussives or suppressants, quiet the brain's cough center.

But if your cough is productive (wet and thick) your doctor will want you to use an expectorant. If your medicine contains an expectorant to promote the coughing up of secretions, however, don't expect it to make your cough go away. It's not designed to do that.

Most cough preparations have two components to help reduce your cough: a syrup and the active drug. While most people think that the thicker cough syrup is the better product, the truth is that syrup components of cough preparations are almost all equally effective, and the thickness of the product doesn't affect the cough suppression, according to Don Bolser, an expert in the cough reflex and assistant professor of physiological sciences at the University of Florida College of Veterinary Medicine. If you want a cough suppressant that doesn't make you tired, look for preparations containing only dextromethorphan; the dose should include 15 mg. or more to suppress your cough.

One of the most common expectorants found in cough medicines is guainfenesin. In the past, experts recommended guainfenesin to thin and loosen mucus in your lungs. But today researchers believe guainfenesin doesn't really do that much for you. Pediatrician Michael Smith M.D., who conducted a comprehensive review of cold medicines, could find only one study on guainfenesin that he believed was scientifically valid—and that study showed guainfenesin did not thin or loosen mucus. Guainfenesin just doesn't work for a cough, according to pharmacy professor Leslie Hendeles at the University of Florida in Gainesville, who testified before Congress about the ingredient's ineffectiveness. "They are supposed to loosen mucus, but they are generally ineffective," writes Dr. Edward Garrity, Jr., director of the Pulmonary Function Lab at the Loyola University Medical Center, in *House Calls: How Doctors Treat Themselves.*

DECONGESTANTS (TOPICAL AND ORAL)

ORAL: *ephedrine oxymetazoline*   *phenylephrine xylometazoline*
         phenylpropanolamine   *pseudoephedrine*

TOPICAL: *nasal sprays (various ingredients:*
          Afrin Spray, 4-Way Nasal Spray,
          Neo- Synephrine)

As soon as you come down with a cold, your body releases a host of chemicals in your nose that makes the blood vessels swell. Since there's more blood flow in your nose per cubic centimeter than even in your brain, you'll notice this swelling right away. Your nose will feel stuffy and congested.

Oral decongestants can be a less-than-optimal choice because they will work to reduce the constriction not just in your nose, but all over your body. They also rev up your central nervous system, making you feel like you've just drunk a quart of coffee; you'll feel nervous, restless, and wakeful. They may cause tremor and palpitations, and aren't a good choice for anyone with heart disease. For these reasons, if you insist on a decongestant many experts prefer nasal sprays to oral products, because they work faster than pills and only reduce constriction in the nose. Phenylephrine lasts for 4 hours and oxymetazoline lasts 8 to 12 hours. There is a down side to these nose drops and sprays, however. If you use them for more than three days and then stop, they can cause a rebound effect, making you feel even more stuffy than you did before you sprayed, according to E.J. Carstensen, M.D., a family physician at the Clinical Nutrition Center in Denver, Colorado. For this reason, they should be taken for as short a period of time as possible.

Because decongestants can raise blood pressure and make you feel jittery, they may not be a good choice if you have severe high blood pressure, you're sensitive to caffeine, or you're taking a prescription drug called monoamine oxidase inhibitors (used in some antidepressants and migraine drugs).

If the rebound effect makes you determined to use decongestant pills, choose pseudoephedrine; it won't boost your blood pressure as much as phenylpropanolamine, the second-most popular decongestant and the main ingredient in some diet pills. Phenylpropanolamine's tendency to raise blood pressure is so pronounced that some experts want it to be taken off the market because of the danger to those with high blood pressure.

Basically, decongestants are all mild stimulants and may interfere with sleeping. "Given the choice, I choose sleep over having an open nose," says Dr. Carstensen.

A decongestant can help shrink swollen blood vessels that block airways in the nose and sinuses, says Dr. Gwaltney. Small amounts of oral or topical decongestants are found in many over-the-counter cold remedies, available in tablet or nose-drop form. They are often used to treat upper respiratory tract infections, especially in those people who are susceptible to middle ear or sinus infections.

THROAT SPRAYS / LOZENGES

If you've got a sore throat, you may notice that some multi-symptom products claim to ease the pain—but if they do, it's only because the medicine contains a decongestant that stops postnasal drip, which can be irritating to sensitive throat tissue. But remember that throats often become sore not because of postnasal drip but because the throat is infected or irritated because of coughing. Drugs designed to stop postnasal drip won't affect the throat infection or soothe the irritation.

If you must use a sore throat medicine, use a throat spray or lozenge that contains a topical anesthetic that works by temporarily deadening nerve endings.

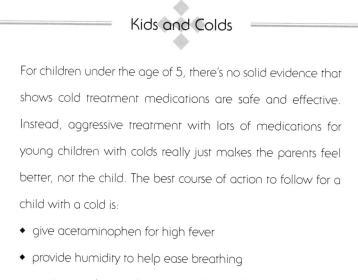

Kids and Colds

For children under the age of 5, there's no solid evidence that shows cold treatment medications are safe and effective. Instead, aggressive treatment with lots of medications for young children with colds really just makes the parents feel better, not the child. The best course of action to follow for a child with a cold is:

- give acetaminophen for high fever

- provide humidity to help ease breathing

- suction out the nasal passages after instilling a few drops of saline solution

- give plenty of fluids to offset dehydration and loosen mucus

- give chicken soup for immune-boosting properties

- provide reassurance

Getting Past the Advertising Hype

There are no standards when it comes to figuring out what the hype really means on the front of a box of cold medication. Words like "fast-acting," "extra-strength," or "pediatric formula" may mean different things to different companies.

Keep in mind that a "maximum strength" drug often just provides a bigger dose than similar products made by the same company. But if you're dealing with a multi-symptom formula, it's hard to figure out which ingredient is stronger.

The only way to really understand the differences is to study the ingredient lists on the boxes, comparing ingredients and dosages to other similar products. But keep in mind that the fine print on all those boxes is often just a way for the company to position their product to make it stand out from the competition.

As you can see, most drugs that supposedly treat cold symptoms just don't work—and they may cause a host of unwanted side effects. That's why going natural in most cases is the best path to getting rid of your cold symptoms. For example, several studies have found that taking one 500 mg. tablet of vitamin C four times a day can lessen both the symptoms and the duration of a cold. Studies of zinc lozenges show that they halve the duration of a typical cold, and the herb echinacea may prevent or shorten the duration of colds caused by some varieties of virus.

In the chapters that follow, you'll learn about a whole host of natural, effective ways to treat each symptom of your cold, without resorting to over-the-counter medications or prescription drugs.

CHAPTER TWO

21 Simple Ways
to Prevent a Cold

E ALL KNOW HOW it starts: Your throat feels a little scratchy, your eyes start to water, your nose runs. All you can think about is crawling into bed with a box of tissues, a bowl of chicken soup, and a big, fluffy comforter. This year, Americans will come down with 500 million colds, and each and every one of them will be a little different. As every parent knows, children younger than age 5 get sick the most—almost once a month. By the time we reach adulthood, our immunity can screen out all but two to four colds a year.

But after all this time, the best medical science has been able to come up with is a sack of expensive medications to treat the symptoms. Neither a cure nor a vaccine for the common cold appears to be coming soon, and there may likely never be one. This is because the viruses behind the common cold vary enormously—you could have a cold every year of your life and still not have come down with all the possible types.

Instead, what we can do is to understand how colds are spread, how to prevent them (it can be done!), and how to utilize safe, natural remedies to ease the discomfort without spending lots of money.

Finding a natural solution to the woes of the common cold is important. We lose millions of days of work and school every year, and spend more than $2 billion on over-the-counter and prescription remedies — most of which don't work and can actually make your symptoms worse. By learning how colds are spread, how to treat the symptoms, and how to substitute natural, everyday remedies for expensive and useless drugs, you can try to make the common cold less common.

What Is a Cold?

A cold is a viral infection, one of at least 200 different types. Cold season begins in the fall and continues throughout the spring; tropical areas tend to encourage cold viruses during the rainy months. Cold viruses are found throughout the world, and they infect only humans.

Different types of viruses proliferate at different times; in the fall and late spring, a cold may be caused by one of the more than 100 types of rhinoviruses. These are the most common villains, and appear to be related to crowding indoors, school openings, and seasonal variations, according to Dr. Lynn C. Kratcha at the Minot Center for Family Medicine in Minot, North Dakota. Between December and May, several types of coronaviruses are responsible for most colds. Besides these two types of viruses — rhinoviruses and coronaviruses — colds may also be caused by parainfluenza, RSV, adenovirus, enterovirus, and influenza. All of these viruses seem to be able to change their characteristics from one season to the next.

Colds are considered to be upper respiratory infections, which means they are limited to your nose and throat. Symptoms will include a stuffy or congested nose, sneezing, sore and scratchy throat, cough, headache, runny eyes, and sometimes a low fever. Viruses that attack the lower respiratory tract — the windpipe, bronchial tubes, and lungs — are more serious but less common, and are responsible for pneumonia and bronchitis, among other respiratory conditions. The symptoms of a cold (scratchy throat, runny nose, and congestion) aren't caused by the virus itself, but are the result of your immune system's fight to get rid of the invader.

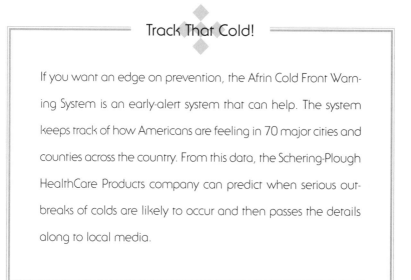

Track That Cold!

If you want an edge on prevention, the Afrin Cold Front Warning System is an early-alert system that can help. The system keeps track of how Americans are feeling in 70 major cities and counties across the country. From this data, the Schering-Plough HealthCare Products company can predict when serious outbreaks of colds are likely to occur and then passes the details along to local media.

Life Cycle of the Common Cold

In a healthy body, you'll find a film of mucus lining your nose and throat; tiny hairs called cilia move this mucus from your sinuses and throat to your stomach. As the mucus is moved along, it traps harmful bacteria and viruses and carries them along to the stomach, where they are broken down by acids. A healthy mucous membrane can snag germs trapped in your nose and throat, and breathe, cough, or sneeze them back out. The mucus around your tonsils and adenoids can trap these germs, where they can be destroyed by the immune system. If you're less than healthy, the mucous membranes in your nose will be either too thick (you'll have a stuffy nose and congested throat) or too thin (runny nose). The germs won't be cleared away.

Once the viruses enter the nose, they set up housekeeping in the mucus layer of the nose and throat, attaching themselves to cells found there. The viruses drill holes in the cell membranes, inserting their own genetic material to enter the cells. Soon the virus takes over and forces the cells to pump out thousands of new little virus particles.

In response to this invasion, the body's immune system swings into action. Injured cells in the nose and throat release chemicals called prostaglandins, which trigger inflammation and attract infection-fighting white blood cells. (Your throat will begin to feel scratchy and swollen.) Tiny blood vessels stretch, which allows spaces to open up and specialized white cells to enter. Body temperature rises and histamine is released (you get a fever). This steps up the production of mucus in the nose, trapping and removing viral particles. (Your nose starts to run.)

All of this activity comes at a price, of course — the unpleasant symptoms you experience as a cold. Actually, by the time you start feeling badly, your body has already been fighting the invader for a day or two. When you're catching a cold, you probably feel fine. It's not until you're getting better that you feel awful.

As the nose and throat stimulate the extra mucus production, it irritates the throat and triggers a cough. Cold viruses are also responsible for congestion in the sinuses.

Because the symptoms of a cold are actually caused by your body's attempt at healing itself, there are times when you should not interfere. It's best to let a fever below 102 degrees F burn itself out, since your body heat will also help you burn up bacteria and toxins. Nausea is your body's way of letting your system heal by stopping food intake. And that mucus from your runny nose is a good way of getting rid of germs.

The good news: After one bout with a particular virus, you will develop an immunity to that precise virus. This is why adults have fewer colds than young children, and why the oldest Americans have the fewest colds of all.

How a Cold Is Transmitted

You cannot catch a cold by sitting in a draft, getting your feet wet, or going outside without a jacket, according to Dr. Bennett Lorber, section chief of Infectious Diseases at Temple University in Philadelphia. It isn't passed along by kissing, either, according to leading virologist Elliot Dick, Ph.D., chief of the Respiratory Virus Research Lab at the University of Wisconsin. Dr. Dick once blindfolded 13 pairs of volunteers and had them kiss for up to a minute and a half in a sterile room. One volunteer in each pair had been infected with the cold virus; the other had neither the cold nor antibodies to the virus. Only one of the 13 cold-free volunteers came down with the cold.

The reason is that cold viruses don't travel mouth to mouth, but hand to nose, according to Jack M. Gwaltney, Jr., chief of epidemiology and virology at the University of Virginia Medical School. Because the cold viruses are so specific, Dr. Gwaltney says, you can only get a cold if the virus travels high up inside your nose, in the nasopharynx. A cold virus can only reach this area by touch, or (less often) through the air. One study found that even a very brief contact with a contaminated hand—as quick as a 10-second touch—led to transmission of virus in 20 of 28 cases.

While cooling the body doesn't seem to bring on a cold, fatigue, stress, and anything else that weakens the body's immune system can influence your susceptibility. You can catch a cold from other people around you who have colds, or from the things they use or touch: faucets, phones, doorknobs, light switches, straps on busses or subways, office equipment. A virus can survive for many hours on these objects, unless someone washes it off with alcohol, a household disinfectant, or hot, sudsy water.

If you touch one of these contaminated objects and then touch your nose, eyes or mouth, you'll get the virus. Once the virus is on your hands, you can expose others as well by shaking hands with them or by touching other things that they touch.

Cold viruses are not carried very far through the air, however. If someone with a cold sneezes across the room, you won't come down with the cold too—but if someone should cough or sneeze right into your face, you could.

Once you become infected, you can pass on the virus to others from 24 hours before symptoms appear until five days after the cold starts. You're most infectious for the first three days from the time when the first symptoms show up, according to Dr. Gwaltney. Young children are infectious for a longer period of time (up to three weeks), since it takes their immune systems longer to fight off the virus. It may not seem practical, but if you have a cold, you should do everyone a favor and stay home. While most adults feel that they should force themselves to go to work if they have a cold, in fact it would be much better for everyone if you would isolate yourself while you have a cold to decrease the spread of the virus.

If you smoke or live in a polluted atmosphere, your chances of coming down with a cold are higher. This is because air pollution and the nicotine and tars in tobacco smoke can irritate the lining of the throat, making it easier for a cold virus to enter your cells and cause an infection, according to Ira W. Gabrielson, M.D., M.P.H., professor and chair of the department of Community and Preventive Medicine at the Medical College of Pennsylvania. This irritation can also prolong the length of the infection. This is why people who live in heavily polluted areas, who smoke, or live with smokers have more colds and have them longer than those who don't.

Complications

A cold usually lasts for about 10 days, although it can range from three days to several weeks. If 10 days have passed and you still feel ill, it's time to call a doctor. Don't wait that long if your face starts to swell, or your teeth become extremely sensitive, because these symptoms can signal a bacterial infection in the sinuses or middle ear. When the sinuses become clogged with nasal secretions, they may become infected with bacteria. While antibiotics won't touch a cold, they will be effective in treating this secondary bacterial infection.

Colds also may trigger asthma attacks in those who suffer with this condition. In children, colds may also lead to middle ear infections, the most common complication of colds. Pneumonia may set in at the end of a cold; if you suddenly develop a fever after the symptoms seem to be going away, see a doctor.

Is It a Cold, Flu, or Allergy?

One of the most important things to understand is that a cold is not the same as the flu. Head colds are just what they say they are — limited to the head. The flu will affect your entire system. A cold will come on gradually, beginning with a vague feeling of unease: the sore throat may be slight, chills or aches will not be severe, and fever won't usually rise above 100 degrees F. The common cold causes:

+ scratchy throat
+ runny nose
+ itchy eyes

On the other hand, influenza strikes fast and hard, with symptoms that are much more severe than those characterized by a simple cold. And while an allergy may cause a stuffy nose and itchy eyes, it does not cause fever, aches, or pains. The flu causes:

+ nausea
+ vomiting
+ diarrhea
+ high fever (from 101°F to 104°F)
+ body aches, especially in the back
+ chills
+ eye pain
+ dry cough
+ light sensitivity
+ headache

Allergies share a few symptoms with colds, but they have significant differences. If your cold seems to be hanging on for months, it could be an allergy. Chances are, your symptoms may get worse if you smell smoke, perfume, tobacco, or some other irritant. Winter allergies (known as perennial allergic rhinitis) cause:

- itchy eyes
- itchy, runny, stuffy nose
- itchy throat
- postnasal drip
- cough
- sneezing
- season-long symptoms

By being careful, it really is possible to stop the spread of colds, even if you're living in a household where others are sick. This is particularly important because studies show that the biggest threat is not the stranger sneezing or hacking next to you on the bus. In order to break through your body's defenses—hair, mucus, and other barriers in the human nose—viruses must attack in huge numbers in order to successfully cause a cold. Most of the time, according to Dr. Dick, a brief encounter with a sick stranger won't put you at risk, even if you're sitting in a doctor's office filled with sick patients for 10 or 20 minutes.

You will have a much better chance of staying healthy during cold season if you follow the guidelines in this chapter.

Don't Touch Your Nose or Eyes!

The most important factor in reducing the transmission of colds is to keep your hands away from your nose and eyes, according to Dr. Gwaltney. By scratching your nose or rubbing your eyes with a virus-infected hand, the virus can easily be inhaled higher up in the nose, or enter the nasopharynx through the tear ducts of the eyes. According to Dr. Gwaltney's studies, most people touch their nose or eyes about once every three hours. It's best if you can manage not to touch your nose or eyes, but if you must, use a knuckle, not your fingertip.

Wash Your Hands

Since it's hard to train yourself not to touch your face, it's a good idea to wash your hands frequently, according to Dr. Gwaltney. Since most folks touch their nose or eyes often, being around a person with a cold means that in all likelihood, you'll get virus on your hands.

If you already have a cold, it's also important to wash your hands often, since you are even more likely to be wiping, blowing, scratching, or touching your nose.

You don't necessarily need an antibacterial soap (one that has triclosan or triclocarban). They are safe and will get rid of bacteria or viruses on your hands—but so will a good scrubbing with ordinary soap or detergent. Washing your hands vigorously with soap and water for 20 seconds will remove the virus. If you don't have ready access to a sink, disposable towelettes are a good alternative.

Try to wash your hands:

- after sneezing or coughing
- before eating
- after wiping, blowing, or touching your nose
- after using the toilet

Keep Your Sneezes to Yourself

Remember not to sneeze or cough directly in anyone's face. Use disposable tissues instead of cloth handkerchiefs when coughing, sneezing, or blowing your nose, and throw them away immediately after using. Remember that a used tissue lying around is filled with virus just waiting to be passed on to someone else.

Disinfect Your Home

In addition to washing your hands and refraining from touching your face, it's also a good idea to disinfect areas likely to be contaminated with germs, such as door handles, telephones, light switches, and so on.

Take Vitamin C

While the use of vitamin C to prevent and treat colds is still controversial, there are many doctors and researchers who do believe that vitamin C is effective in preventing a cold as well as treating its symptoms. According to Dr. Dick, one 500 mg. tablet four times a day is enough to lessen a cold's symptoms and duration. And Andrew Weil, M.D., well-known physician and author, believes that vitamin C is a good way to prevent colds.

Don't Forget Vitamins A and B

Vitamin A can help keep the mucous membranes strong, boosting the body's defense mechanisms. Vitamin B complex can help balance the nerves and endocrine system, and all the B vitamins are excellent for stress, which can weaken the immune system.

Take Echinacea to Boost Your Immune System

Several German studies have suggested that the herb echinacea appears to be a mild stimulant of the immune system that may help fend off colds. Researchers believe it increases the levels of the naturally-occurring antiviral substance interferon, in addition to a blood protein related to the immune system. It also boosts the production of immune cells in bone marrow, the thymus, and the spleen. Scientists have identified chemicals that boost the immune system and counteract inflammation in both the root and other parts of the echinacea plant. Moreover, other studies have recently identified a number of antioxidant compounds in the echinacea plant.

The plant appears in a wide variety of herbal preparations. Derived from roots and other parts of the purple coneflower, the processed native American plant can be found as a fresh juice, tablet, capsule, concentrated drops, tinctures, or extracts. If you take echinacea in its liquid form, you should expect to feel a slight numbing sensation on your tongue. It is often combined with goldenseal, elderberry, vitamin C, and zinc.

In order for it to be effective, you need to take echinacea at the very first sign of a cold, according to Mark Mayell, author of *Off the Shelf Natural Health* and coauthor of *The Natural Health First-Aid Guide* and *52 Steps to Natural Health*. If you wait until you're coughing and sniffling, you've waited too long.

Herbalists recommend that if you want to take echinacea as a stimulant to the immune system, you should take it cyclically, not constantly—every other week, for example. This is because its effect appears to fade when used on a daily basis for longer than eight weeks.

Echinacea is an extremely safe herb and is not known to cause any side effects. However, if you're allergic to other plants in this family —including sunflowers, daisies, or dandelions—take only a small dose at first. Even so, allergic reactions to this herb are very rare.

Try Garlic, A Powerful Healer

Garlic in a capsule, tablet, or supplement form, taken two to four times a day, may help with the common cold, according to Dr. Mark Blumenthal, founder and executive director of the American Botanical Council. Garlic has been used for its health-giving properties for thousands of years.

A member of the lily family, it is among the oldest cultivated plants still in existence and has been touted in an incredible range of folk remedies guaranteed to protect against everything from werewolves to insect bites. In the past 20 years, more than 2,400 scientific studies have looked at its constituents and its effects on health. Recent research studies have found that it can boost immunity and prevent digestive ailments, among a host of other health-giving properties. A complex substance, garlic contains amino acids, vitamins and trace minerals, flavonoids, enzymes, and at least 200 other compounds. The source of its antiviral and antioxidant properties is believed to be its sulfur compounds, which are rarely found in any other plants.

Drink Plenty of Fluids

Be sure to get from eight to ten glasses of liquid a day, according to Robert Cooper, Ph.D., president of the Center for Health & Fitness in Bemidji, Minnesota. Drinking fluids keeps the throat moist and helps trap viruses that find their way into the nose or throat. Drinking a liquid diet of clear broths, herbal teas, and juices for a day or two may help to prevent a cold. Or try ginger root or peppermint tea, with ginger, honey, lemon, cayenne, cinnamon, and peppermint.

Drink Cold-Preventing Astragalus Tea

This sweet, pleasant-tasting Chinese herb packs a powerful immune-strengthening wallop, according to herbalists, which can boost immune activity in a variety of ways. For example, astragalus can boost white blood cell activity and step up the production of antibodies. While it is considered to be a "warming" herb according to traditional Chinese medicine and therefore not something that should be taken during a cold, it is an excellent preventive tonic.

Dried astragalus root and extracts are available at many herb and natural food stores. Extracts made from astragalus can be used instead of tea. If you want to make your own strong astragalus tea in the Chinese manner, follow this simple recipe:

ASTRAGALUS TEA

2 ounces dried astragalus root
1½ cups water

Simmer ingredients in covered pot for an hour. Strain, then save the liquid and the herb. Simmer the herb a second time in 1½ cups of fresh water for 30 minutes. Strain, then discard the herb. Combine liquid from both batches and drink one cup of this tea in the morning and again in the evening to prevent a cold from coming on.

Foods and Drinks to Avoid

Certain foods and beverages will inhibit your body's ability to fight off a cold. Follow these guidelines to keep your immune system strong:

1. Drop dairy products from your diet if you're in danger of catching a cold, recommends Dr. Blumenthal. Some researchers believe dairy products unnecessarily thicken mucous membranes, which can worsen cold symptoms.

2. Avoid sweets. All forms of sugar interfere with the infection-fighting white blood cells. As infected cells die, they attract these white blood cells to digest the invading germs; if you've been downing sweets, the white blood cells won't have the power to do the job. Even a few cans of soda can cut the effectiveness of these helper cells in half.

3. Avoid alcohol. Like sugar, alcohol interferes with the effectiveness of infection-fighting white blood cells, particularly if you drink it every day.

Cold-Preventing Tea Recipes

Here's a good recipe to prevent the onset of cold symptoms, as recommended by many herbalists:

Add one dropperful of commercially-prepared tincture of goldenseal and echinacea to either chamomile or ginger tea. Drink a cup four times a day when you are at risk for getting a cold.⁺

You can also take echinacea and goldenseal by themselves, adding a dropper of each to a cup of water and drinking four times a day.

CHAMOMILE TEA

Brew chamomile tea with a tea bag, or brew a teaspoon of dried flowers in a cup of steaming hot water for three minutes before straining.

GINGER TEA

Remove the skin of a 2-inch piece of gingerroot. Cut off thin slices. Brew in steaming hot water for 10 minutes before straining.

CAUTION: Most health practitioners recommend against taking echinacea or goldenseal on an ongoing basis because of their powerful effects. Use these herbs only when you are really threatened with a cold.

Mellow Out

There is a definite link between emotions and infections, according to studies reported in the *New England Journal of Medicine*. In one study by Sheldon Cohen, Ph.D., professor of psychology at Carnegie-Mellon University in Pittsburgh, a high level of psychological and emotional stress lowers your resistance to viral infections, and nearly doubles your chances of getting a cold. A number of other studies have produced similar results. According to Bernie Siegel, M.D., author of several best-selling books including *Love, Medicine, and Miracles* and *How to Live Between Office Visits*, humor, love, time alone, and loving your life are all good ways to boost your immune system and prevent a cold.

Relax!

New evidence suggests that practicing relaxation techniques and positive imagery can shorten the duration of a viral infection — sometimes within an hour or so — by boosting the action of the body's immune system. Meditation has been shown to increase the production of immunoglobulin A (IgA), an antibody that helps fend off colds. Here are eight ways to relax:

- meditation
- biofeedback
- visualization
- yoga
- relaxation tapes
- listening to soothing music
- watching fish
- petting your dog or cat

Some experts recommend that the "stress vitamins" — the water soluble vitamins B complex and C with bioflavonoids — can offset environmental and emotional stress.

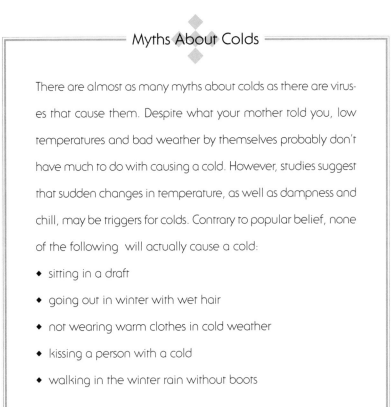

Myths About Colds

There are almost as many myths about colds as there are viruses that cause them. Despite what your mother told you, low temperatures and bad weather by themselves probably don't have much to do with causing a cold. However, studies suggest that sudden changes in temperature, as well as dampness and chill, may be triggers for colds. Contrary to popular belief, none of the following will actually cause a cold:

- sitting in a draft
- going out in winter with wet hair
- not wearing warm clothes in cold weather
- kissing a person with a cold
- walking in the winter rain without boots

There are also a number of old folk remedies that just don't work in treating symptoms of a cold. These include:

- breathing steam up into the nose
- feed a cold, starve a fever (you should feed both)
- taking antibiotics

Laugh a Little

Humor also helps to prevent illness. Well-known laughter advocate Norman Cousins discusses the health-giving properties of laughter in his classic book, *Anatomy of an Illness*. In one study by psychologist Kathleen Dillon, Ph.D., at Western New England College in Springfield, Massachusetts, researchers discovered that levels of protective chemicals, such as IgA, can be increased with laughter. One group of volunteers in this study watched comedies, while a second group watched documentaries. The IgA levels in the first group rose significantly; the levels of IgA in the second group stayed the same.

Humidify Your Home

Studies suggest that the relative humidity of the air you breathe may affect how many colds you get. During the winter, there is both a sharp increase in the number of colds and the start of winter heating, which lowers humidity in the air. Many heating systems keep the home environments too dry, according to Dr. Gabrielson. This low humidity causes dry throats and noses, which increases the chance of infection.

Your nose, throat, and lungs work best when the air has a relative humidity of about 45 percent. If the air in your house during the winter falls below that level and it becomes too dry, your mucous membranes will dry out. Since dried mucous membranes can't clean themselves, they become more vulnerable to invasion from cold viruses.

To help prevent colds, try running a humidifier in your bedroom to add moisture to the dry air. You may also try keeping the thermostat at 68 degrees F; cooler air can help retain more moisture.

Keep Air Circulating

Good ventilation can also help disperse germs and hinder the spread of colds, according to Dr. Dick. Keep windows open at home, and if there's a forced-air ventilation system at work, make sure it's working

Humidifier Health

Using a humidifier during the winter can help prevent colds. But to prevent mold-related allergies, it's imperative that you use the device correctly. If the air becomes too humid, or the machine isn't properly cleaned, mold and dust mites can multiply. This can cause allergies which may be mistaken for colds.

When using a humidifier, follow these simple guidelines in your home:

◆ Don't let the humidity rise above 30 percent.

◆ Clean the water reservoir daily with a vinegar
  solution.

◆ Limit the number of plants in your home.

◆ Empty the refrigerator drip pan frequently.

◆ Keep firewood outside your house.

◆ Use exhaust fans in the bathroom and kitchen.

◆ Vent clothes dryer outside your house.

◆ Regularly wash bathroom walls, fixtures, and shower
  curtains with anti-mold solutions.

◆ Use only washable mats (not carpet) in the bathroom.

◆ Don't put carpet directly on a concrete floor.

well. It should bring fresh air from the outside, and withdraw stale indoor air. If you have electric baseboard heat or radiators, use fans to circulate the air.

The closed circulation systems of airplanes are another potential danger for the transmission of colds, according to Dr. Siegel, in *How to Live Between Office Visits*. This is because the recirculated air in a pressurized cabin distributes viruses throughout the cabin to everybody, while drying out mucous membranes that would normally trap viruses. If you must travel on a plane carrying sick passengers, you're more likely to come down with a cold yourself. To combat the low humidity of on-plane air, Dr. Siegel recommends drinking lots of fluids on planes — and avoiding alcohol, which can dehydrate your body. He also notes that it's usually healthier in first class than in the back of the plane, depending on how many people are on board. Some experts recommend that you drink at least 8 ounces of water for each hour you spend on a plane to rehydrate the nose.

Isolate Personal Articles

If there are cold germs circulating in your household, don't share your eating or drinking utensils with others (especially babies). Use a separate set of towels and washcloths, and change your bedding more often. Actually, bedding should be changed more often for everyone, healthy or sick, during the winter months to help cut down on virus transmission.

Change Your Toothbrush Often

Since viruses can live on many different objects, some experts recommend that you buy a new toothbrush when you recover from a cold. While it's not likely that rhinovirus (the most common cold virus) can make you sick by hitching a ride on your toothbrush — they must get into your nose to cause a cold — viruses such as the enterovirus (found in the stomach/intestines) can occasionally cause a cold. To be safe, experts suggest you replace your toothbrush every three months—and never share a toothbrush with anyone!

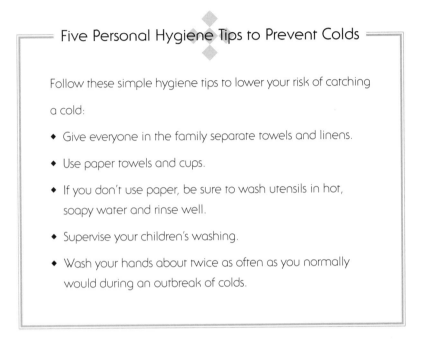

Five Personal Hygiene Tips to Prevent Colds

Follow these simple hygiene tips to lower your risk of catching a cold:

♦ Give everyone in the family separate towels and linens.

♦ Use paper towels and cups.

♦ If you don't use paper, be sure to wash utensils in hot, soapy water and rinse well.

♦ Supervise your children's washing.

♦ Wash your hands about twice as often as you normally would during an outbreak of colds.

Take a Hot Bath

Hot baths several times a day using herbal oils such as those containing peppermint or wintergreen may help head off an incipient cold, according to Dr. Blumenthal.

Dress Warmly

According to traditional Chinese medicine, a virus enters the body via the head, neck, and chest areas, as well as the feet. If you cover those parts of the body and keep them warm with silk, wool, or cotton next to the skin, you may ward off colds.

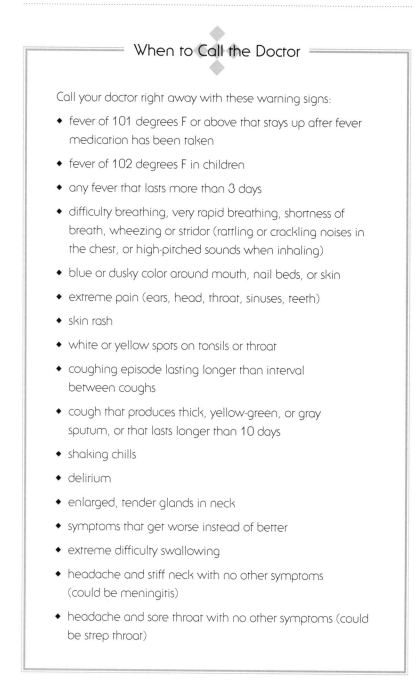

When to Call the Doctor

Call your doctor right away with these warning signs:

- fever of 101 degrees F or above that stays up after fever medication has been taken

- fever of 102 degrees F in children

- any fever that lasts more than 3 days

- difficulty breathing, very rapid breathing, shortness of breath, wheezing or stridor (rattling or crackling noises in the chest, or high-pitched sounds when inhaling)

- blue or dusky color around mouth, nail beds, or skin

- extreme pain (ears, head, throat, sinuses, teeth)

- skin rash

- white or yellow spots on tonsils or throat

- coughing episode lasting longer than interval between coughs

- cough that produces thick, yellow-green, or gray sputum, or that lasts longer than 10 days

- shaking chills

- delirium

- enlarged, tender glands in neck

- symptoms that get worse instead of better

- extreme difficulty swallowing

- headache and stiff neck with no other symptoms (could be meningitis)

- headache and sore throat with no other symptoms (could be strep throat)

Treat Your Body Well

It's important to treat your body well if you want to prevent colds. Plenty of exercise and sufficient rest will improve your circulation, lymphatic system, organs, and emotions. In one study, volunteers who exercised regularly showed improved immune function, and only half as many days of cold symptoms. But remember that too much of a good thing can be harmful—those who exercised too strenuously depressed their immune systems, and actually increased their risk of getting colds, according to David Nieman, D.H.Sc., professor of health education at Appalachian State University in Boone, North Carolina. Any moderate noncompetitive exercise can work, up to an hour at a time. Experts recommend exercise several times a week —not every day.

In the Next Chapter

In the next chapter, you'll learn lots of natural ways recommended by experts to get rid of that overall sick feeling caused by the common cold.

36 Ways to Get Rid of
That Overall Sick Feeling

HILE THIS BOOK treats each symptom of the common cold separately, there are also many natural treatments for generalized symptoms of a cold—that sick feeling, usually accompanied by a sense of malaise.

Herbs have long been used successfully to treat general cold and flu symptoms because of their ability to stimulate immune function and fight viruses and inflammation. In this chapter, you'll learn about them as well as other effective natural treatments for that overall sick feeling.

Try Lomatium (Lomatia) for a Boost

This relatively unknown herb is an antiviral and an immune system stimulant, according to John Hibbs, N.D., of Seattle, Washington. Dr. Hibbs believes it is the most effective flu remedy among all the herbs, and says he has observed full recovery from common cold symptoms on many occasions within 24 to 48 hours of taking lomatium. Take a lomatium tincture mixed with the herbs ligustium and echinacea three to four times a day, with plenty of liquids, lots of rest, and no alcohol or sugar. Although this herb is sometimes hard to find, look in health food stores, herb outlets, and specialty garden centers. See Appendix B for suppliers of hard-to-find herbs and seeds.

❖❖❖ CAUTION: Lomatium can cause an itchy measles-like rash on the skin of sensitive people or those who take too large a dose.

Consider Echinacea, a Powerful Healing Herb

A member of the daisy family, this native American herb is derived from the roots of *Echinacea angustifolia* or the leaves and roots of *E. purpurea*. It was used for many years by Native Americans, who understood its healing properties, and is very popular today throughout Europe. Echinacea, an anti-inflammatory and anti-infectious agent, can be a real help in treating generalized cold symptoms, according to Centerville, Ohio physician John H. Boyles, Jr., of Dayton Ear, Nose, and Throat Surgeons in Centerville, Ohio.

It stimulates white blood cells (part of your immune system), acts as a mild antibiotic, stimulates the production of healthy tissue, inhibits tumors, promotes general cellular immunity, and has antiviral and anti-inflammatory properties. Scientists also suspect that it increases the ability of the body to produce white blood cells that help destroy bacteria and viruses. It also encourages the body to produce its own antiviral weapon, interferon, a substance that cold-infected cells release in tiny amounts as they die. Interferon signals white blood cells that an infection is in the body, and summons their help.

At the first sign of a cold, take 15 to 20 drops of a combination of echinacea and goldenseal four times a day, according to Alan Cohen, M.D., medical director of Harmony Health Care in Milford, Connecticut. It's important to take echinacea at the first sneeze. Many people take it as a tincture (an alcohol extract) because it is the most potent form.

✦ CAUTION: Do not take echinacea for long periods of time; stop taking this herb when your symptoms subside.

Sip Goldenseal, a Natural Antibiotic

Goldenseal contains a powerful natural antibiotic known as berberine, a substance that may stimulate the immune system and is often combined with echinacea as a cold treatment. It activates macrophages, the immune cells that engulf and destroy bacteria, viruses, and other foreign substances. As with echinacea, it should be used only to fight an illness and not taken on a regular basis.

For an invigorating drink and cold treatment, try this combination tea:

ECHINACEA/GOLDENSEAL TEA

1 dropper of tincture of echinacea
1 dropper of tincture of goldenseal
chamomile or ginger tea

Brew chamomile tea either with a tea bag or by brewing a teaspoon of the dried flowers in a cup of steaming hot water for three minutes before straining. Brew ginger tea by removing the skin of a 2-inch piece of gingerroot, cutting off thin slices, and brewing them in steaming hot water for 10 minutes before straining. Drink a cup of this tea 4 times a day when you have a cold.

✦ CAUTION: Most natural health practitioners do not recommend taking echinacea or goldenseal on an ongoing basis. Reserve these herbs for times when you have a cold. Do not take goldenseal during pregnancy.

Take Astragalus for Your Immune System

This Chinese medicinal herb has long been valued in Asia as an immune system enhancer and can help improve immune function, according to well-known physician and best-selling author Andrew Weil, M.D., associate director of the Division of Social Perspectives in Medicine at the University of Arizona College of Medicine. Dr. Weil suggests taking two capsules of astragalus three times a day for the duration of the illness.

Or you can drink it as a tincture (1–1 ½ teaspoons of tincture three times a day) or drink 250–500 mg. of powdered herb in hot water three times a day. If you prefer soup, try this:

ASTRAGALUS SOUP RECIPE I

astragalus	whole bulb of garlic
cayenne pepper	minced fresh ginger

Combine ingredients and heat to simmer. Drink as often as you wish.

ASTRAGALUS SOUP RECIPE II

several slices astragalus root	⅓ cup brown basmati rice
handful fresh/dried shiitake and maitake mushrooms	2 cups sliced vegetables: carrots, celery, onions, etc.
bulb peeled garlic	olive oil
sliced burdock root	light miso
2 inches sliced fresh gingerroot	chopped scallions

Simmer first 6 ingredients in 8 cups of water for an hour. Sauté sliced vegetables in olive oil, add to soup, and simmer for another half hour. Remove astragalus, slice mushrooms and remove any hard stems. Add miso to taste and garnish with chopped scallions.

Sip Elderberry Extract for Quick Relief

For general cold symptoms, try elderberry extract (sambucal) in lozenge form, according to Donald J. Carrow, M.D., of Clearwater, Florida. If used when the first symptoms appear, it can short-circuit most colds, he says.

Try Grapefruit Seed Extract, a Natural Antibiotic

Use grapefruit seed extract both orally and as a gargle, advises Paul Dunn, M.D., of Oak Park, Illinois. The extract has both an antibiotic and antiviral effect. It can be found in most health food stores.

Take Olive Leaf Extract

To counter generalized cold symptoms, take one 500 mg. tablet of olive leaf extract four times a day, according to Cliff Arrington, M.D., of Kealakekua, Hawaii.

Try a Livicera-Forsythia Combination for Early Symptoms

For early symptoms of the common cold, take between 12 and 24 pellets of TCB 16 (livicera/forsythia combination) and repeat as needed during the first 24 hours, according to Richard Bahr, M.D., of Centerville, Ohio. Dr. Bahr estimates the cure rate for this treatment to be at least 75 percent.

Take Yin Chiao, an Effective Chinese Cold Remedy

According to Chinese medicine, a cold is an invasion of the body by the elements wind and heat. A formula known as *Yin Chiao Chieh Tu Pien* expels this wind and heat from the respiratory tract, according to Chinese teachings. Containing primarily honeysuckle and forsythia, it is available from many practitioners of Chinese medicine.

It's enthusiastically endorsed by Harriet Beinfeld, a licensed acupuncturist who practices Chinese medicine in San Francisco, and is a coauthor of *Between Heaven and Earth: A Guide To Chinese Medicine*. At the first sign of a cold, she advises taking 6 tablets of yin chiao every 3 hours.

Eat Garlic, the Multi-Purpose Healer

As soon as you notice signs of a cold or the flu, it's time to turn to garlic, according to Dr. Boyles. The allicin in garlic is the important ingredient, which is why garlic capsules or liquid garlic extract are good choices — both provide higher, more concentrated doses of allicin than you'd get by eating garlic cloves. You can find deodorized garlic capsules in health food outlets. These forms of eating garlic also eliminate that pesky odor problem. If you take garlic capsules, take 10 in the first six hours.

Other experts prefer raw garlic, believing that garlic capsules don't work as well as raw garlic since you must take about 10 capsules to achieve the same results as a single clove. If you opt for raw, eat 2 to 4 cloves daily, finely chopped and swallowed with some water. You could also drink garlic tea.

Remember that allicin — that enzyme that gives garlic its pungent smell — is inactivated by heat. Cooked garlic may be less smelly, but it's also lost most of its medicinal value. For this reason, if you're eating garlic for your health, eat it raw or drink it in a tea. Fresh and powdered garlic have been found to have efficient antibiotic effects, even controlling bacteria that are resistant to commonly-used antibiotics. In some medical studies, garlic has been shown to protect against flu viruses and enhance antibody production.

According to Dr. Kristine Nolfi, M.D., in her book, *My Experiences with Living Food*, if you put a piece of garlic in your mouth on both sides between cheek and teeth at the beginning of a cold, the cold will disappear within a few hours (or at most, within a day). Every so often, release a little garlic juice by digging your teeth into the clove. Replace the clove every two or three hours.

If you're a soup fan, you can try this healing garlic soup, recommended by Annemarie Colbin, founder of the Natural Gourmet Cookery School in New York and author of *Good and Healing*:

GARLIC MISO SOUP

1 head of peeled garlic
1 quart of vegetable stock
1 tablespoon miso (more if desired)

Simmer garlic in stock for 10 minutes. Blend the cloves with one cup of the stock and miso. Return to pot, and season to taste with additional miso if desired.

❖❖ CAUTION: Although garlic is considered very safe, people who use it and are also taking anticoagulants (blood thinners) should be careful since garlic thins the blood.

Sip Cold-Fighting Ginger-Garlic Tea

Dr. Weil makes this strong ginger-garlic tea to fight off colds:

1 teaspoon grated ginger
1 cup water
1 clove crushed garlic
1 tablespoon fresh lemon juice
¼ teaspoon cayenne powder
honey

Simmer ginger in water in covered pot for 5 minutes. Strain. Add garlic, lemon juice, and cayenne powder. Sweeten with honey if desired.

Sniff Herbs for Cold Relief

Aromatherapy is a branch of herbal medicine in which you inhale oils and essences of herbs commonly used to treat health problems. For a good common cold treatment, use aromatherapy by adding these oils to hot bath water:

- 3 drops of lemon oil
- 2 drops of thyme oil
- 2 drops of tea tree oil
- 1 drop of eucalyptus oil

Lie back and inhale deeply.

Watch Your Diet

If you're hungry, eat light foods such as vegetables and fruits, which alkalinize the body and neutralize acidic toxins. Cut out fat, advises Elson Haas, M.D., director of the Marin Clinic of Preventive Medicine and Health Education in San Rafael, California and author of *Staying Healthy with the Seasons*. Since high-fat diets force your immune system to work overtime to prevent heart disease and cancer, this can interfere with its effectiveness in fighting off colds. Moreover, a plant-based diet supports the immune system's fight against illness because plant foods are full of vitamins and minerals necessary for a healthy immune system.

Avoid These Foods and Drinks

All forms of sugar—sucrose, fructose, glucose, honey, and others—interfere with the activity of the infection-fighting white blood cells (the neutrophils), according to Linda Wright, M.D., of Boulder, Colorado. As your cold-infected cells die, they attract these white blood cells to digest the invading microorganisms. But if you've been wolfing down sweets, the white blood cells become lethargic. Even a couple of cans of soda cuts their effectiveness in half.

Also avoid concentrated sweet and hydrogenated oils, or highly processed foods such as potato chips.

While you're at it, stay away from milk, which can seriously stress the immune system and places a burden on the respiratory and digestive systems as well, according to Christiane Northrup, M.D., a Yarmouth, Maine gynecologist. In one recent study, a chemical in milk triggered the release of histamine, which triggers many cold symptoms.

Finally, alcohol is another enemy of white blood cells. If you're getting a cold, cut out alcohol so you don't impair your white blood cell activity.

Eat Your Veggies

Everyone knows that eating generous portions of fruits and vegetables will help keep you healthy. If you're fighting a cold, green and orange vegetables are especially good choices because they provide beta-carotene, according to Dr. Hibbs. The vegetables that are richest in beta-carotene are leafy greens, carrots, and orange squash. During cold and flu season, eat at least one of each every day.

Tap into the Healing Properties of Mushrooms

Certain mushrooms (such as reishitaki and ganoderma) are considered important illness-fighting foods in China and Japan, and may help stimulate the immune system. Mushrooms contain a range of novel compounds not found elsewhere in nature, according to Dr. Weil. He notes that mushrooms are close relatives of molds, from which antibiotics are derived. Try mushrooms raw or added to vegetable or chicken soups.

Drink Fluids

Water can help replace important fluids lost during a cold, according to Robert Snider, M.D., of Massena, New York. If you've got a cold, drink several glasses of pure water a day. In addition, drink a total of at least two quarts of fluid daily (either hot or cold). This is about one glass of juice, water, soda, and so on, every two hours.

Take Vitamins A and C

Probabaly no natural remedy is as well known against the symptoms of a common cold as vitamin C. While still disputed by some scientists, many physicians enthusiastically support the use of large doses of vitamin C to treat cold symptoms. Numerous studies have shown that those who take megadoses of vitamin C (far larger than amounts recommended by the RDA) show reductions in the incidence, severity, and duration of colds.

In addition to fighting viruses and bacteria, vitamin C also boosts the immune system by enhancing white blood cell production and increasing the production of interferon, a group of proteins released by white blood cells that fight viruses. It boosts antibody responses, promotes secretion of thymic hormones, and improves connective tissue.

Well-designed studies suggest that vitamin C, when taken at the first sign of a cold, can reduce symptoms and shorten the duration. The necessary doses are very high and may irritate your stomach or urinary tract. For any cold or flu, vitamin C at a dose of 3 to 6 grams a day for several days at the first sign of a cold supports the immune capacity of the white blood cells, acts as an antihistamine and anti-inflammatory, and promotes healing, according to Richard Junin, M.D., of San Francisco. Take vitamin C to bowel tolerance (until you experience diarrhea) according to Stephen B. Edelson, M.D., of the Environmental and Preventive Health Center of Atlanta. When you do get diarrhea, figure out how many milligrams it took to get the loose stool, and take 75 percent of that daily in three divided doses. The powdered ascorbate form of vitamin C can reduce the chances of your having excess gas or bowel cramping and diarrhea. (High doses can also worsen preexisting gastrointestinal conditions.)

The benefits of vitamin C are augmented by taking vitamin A at doses up to 100,000 IU per day for about a week, according to Dr. Junin. Many doctors believe it is important to take high doses of vitamin A at the same time as the vitamin C, usually for not less than three days but not more than five. Experts believe there is no documented evidence of serious toxicity due to high doses of vitamin A as long as it is used only for a short period of time.

It is important to take vitamin A directly rather than supplementing it with beta-carotene, which is synthesized in the liver to form vitamin A. Trying to synthesize enough vitamin A from beta-carotene would overtax the liver.

In addition, recommends Dr. Junin, you can add zinc in doses up to 100 mg. per day, and 1 to 2 grams of glutamine three times a day.

Drink Vitamin-Rich Juice

If you prefer getting your vitamins the natural way, try drinking orange, tomato, grapefruit, or pineapple juice—at least 5 glasses a day. Studies show "drinking" vitamin C reduces sneezing and coughing in cold sufferers, according to Jeffrey Jahre, M.D., clinical assistant professor of medicine at Temple University School of Medicine in Philadelphia, and chief of the Infectious Diseases Section at St. Luke's Medical Center in Bethlehem, Pennsylvania.

Take Virus-Fighting Monolaurian

This fatty acid is available in capsules and has been shown in research studies to boost the immune system's fight against viruses, according to Timothy Van Ert, M.D., private practitioner and specialist in self-care and preventive medicine in San Francisco and Saratoga, California.

Take 2 capsules of monolaurian 3 times a day with food to treat early cold symptoms, according to Dr. Edelson.

Suck on Zinc for Treating and Preventing Colds

Another important nutrient for maintaining your immune system is zinc, according to recent research. Zinc is a trace element essential for digestion, reproduction, kidney function, diabetes control, taste, and smell. Trials in the 1980s suggested that zinc-based compounds could shorten the duration of colds. Recent reports suggest that particular zinc compounds, if taken as soon as symptoms appear, could stop a cold before it starts because the zinc prevents viruses from attaching themselves to healthy cells.

Experts recommend that you take six zinc lozenges each containing 11.5 mg. a day, for a total of 69 mg., until your symptoms subside. According to Dr. Trevor Delves, consultant biochemist at England's Southampton University, taking large doses of zinc won't be harmful over a short period of time, but he warns that over a long period of time it could interfere with the absorption of copper which can be serious. For prevention, as little as 15 mg. a day helps to bolster the immune system by strengthening the thymus gland.

Some studies suggest that zinc relieves colds only if you start using it right away. The lozenges should be taken after eating to avoid upsetting your stomach, according to zinc researcher Dr. William Halcomb of Mesa, Arizona. If you don't like the taste of the zinc (and it is terrible), Dr. Halcomb recommends that you suck on a peppermint candy at the same time.

Dr. Edelson recommends taking 100 mg. of elemental zinc picolinate daily for 5 days.

Investigate the Ayurvedic Tradition

In India and elsewhere, Ayurvedic practitioners recommend a variety of herbs and dietary guidelines to treat colds. The objective of this type of medicine is to rid the body of indigestible toxins that attract viruses and interfere with the immune process.

To ease your cold symptoms the Ayurvedic way, take 1 to 4 grams

(4 grams is about one rounded teaspoon) of any of these powdered herbs two to three times a day in hot water:

* ginger
* cinnamon
* licorice
* basil
* cloves
* mint

The Ayurvedic diet for colds emphasizes whole grains and steamed vegetables, and recommends that you avoid:

* dairy products
* all animal fats
* oily foods
* nuts
* pastries
* sweet fruit juices

Drinking lots of warm water and ginger tea throughout the day also helps, according to Virender Sodhi, M.D., N.D., director of the American School of Ayurvedic Sciences in Bellevue, Washington.

Slurp Chicken Soup, the Age-Old Remedy

First prescribed by Moses Maimonides in the 12th century, soup made from a fat hen has been treating colds successfully ever since. According to Marvin Sackner, M.D., director of medical services at Mount Sinai Medical Center in Miami Beach, Florida, chicken soup actually does have healing properties and can help cure a cold.

It's also been proven to work better in concert with vegetables than just with the chicken broth alone, according to Stephen Rennard, M.D., chief of pulmonary and critical care medicine at the University of Nebraska Medical Center in Omaha, Nebraska. Dr. Rennard tested plain chicken broth in a test tube and found it somewhat reduced the inflammation-producing activity of white blood cells, suggesting it might ease some cold symptoms. When he added vegetables (onions, sweet potatoes, carrots, turnips, and parsnips), he found the anti-inflammatory effect grew stronger.

Any hot liquid can cut through congestion, but it's much more comforting to sip a bowl of chicken soup than plain water. And it's a good way to get protein-rich nutrients if you don't feel like eating, according to Frederick Ruben, M.D., professor of medicine at the University of Pittsburgh.

Follow this simple recipe:

CHICKEN SOUP

4–5 pounds of chicken

3 carrots (scrubbed or peeled), cut in thirds

2 parsnips (scrubbed), cut in thirds

2 celery stalks with leaves, cut in thirds

1 large onion, cut in half

1 green pepper, cut in half and cleaned out

2 sprigs of dill or ½ teaspoon of dill seeds (optional)

4 parsley sprigs

4 cloves of garlic, crushed

1–2 teaspoons of salt

10 cups of water

Combine chicken, vegetables, water, and salt in a big pot. Wrap dill or seeds, parsley, and garlic in cheesecloth, and add to pot. Bring to boil, clean off scum from the top of the soup, cover and simmer for 2–3 hours. If after three hours the soup doesn't have the flavor you want, add a few chicken bouillon cubes to taste. Remove and reserve chicken and vegetables; refrigerate soup overnight. The next day, remove the top layer of fat from the soup before reheating, skimming the surface with a spoon. Add vegetables and chicken, and heat through.

Explore Homeopathy

Homeopathy works on the theory that substances that can produce the symptoms in question will cure those symptoms by prompting the immune system to action, if taken in tiny doses. Most homeopathic medicines come from plants used in traditional herbal medicine; a few come from animal sources or naturally-occurring chemical compounds. Some medicines—such as mercury and belladonna—are poisonous, but in the superdilute homeopathic doses they are safe when used as recommended. *Although you can buy most of these homeopathic remedies over the counter, it is best to consult with a practitioner who understands the exact use of the many individual homeopathic remedies.*

The most common remedies for the common cold recommended by homeopaths include microdoses of onion (*Allium cepa*), eyebright (*Euphrasia*), salt (*Natrum mur*), monkshood (*Aconite*), wild hops (*Bryonia*), belladonna, and phosphorus.

Still, homeopathy is not universally embraced, and is considered by many mainstream physicians to be little short of quackery. There are about 2,000 homeopaths in the United States, and about half of them are physicians.

U.S. homeopaths typically use the abbreviation "x" to describe a medicine's strength. A potency of 1x means a 1:10 dilution of the original substance; 2x means 1:100, 3x means 1:1000, and so on. Most sold for home use vary in potency from 3x to 30x. Homeopathic medicines aren't simply diluted. They are also shaken vigorously to transfer the medicine's essence to the water used to dilute it. This concept is important, since solutions diluted beyond 24x may not contain even a single molecule of the original solution. Critics say that these extremely dilute solutions are nothing more than water. Homeopaths believe that medicines become stronger as they become more dilute, and that even when enormously dilute their "essence" (or energy) is the same.

Homeopathic medicines usually come in small tablets, beads, or granules onto which the dilute medicine has been placed. Bottles should be tightly capped, away from direct sun and at room temperature. Do not touch the medicine; shake the recommended number of beads or tablets from the bottle into the cap, and place in your mouth without touching them.

How to Find a Homeopathic Practitioner

If you can't find a homeopathic practitioner in your local Yellow Pages, try contacting one of these national organizations:

Homeopathic Educational Services
2124 Kittredge St.
Berkeley, CA 94704

National Center for Homeopathy
801 N. Fairfax, #306
Alexandria, VA 22314

International Foundation for Homeopathy
2366 Eastlake Ave. East, Suite 301
Seattle, WA 98102
(206) 324-8230

Naturopaths (N.D.s) use classical homeopathy as one of their treatments. For more information, contact:

Homeopathic Academy of Naturopathic Physicians
14653 Graves Rd.
Mulion, OR 97042
(503) 829-7326 or (503) 829-7326 (fax)

All homeopathic medicines are sold over-the-counter in health food stores. There have been few reports of adverse reactions.

According to Dr. Andrew Lockie, M.D., in *The Family Guide to Homeopathy*, you should take the remedy that most closely matches your symptoms. Take the dosage recommended on the package every two hours for up to four doses. Again, although you can buy most of these remedies over-the-counter, it is best to consult with a practitioner who understands the exact use of the many individual homeopathic remedies.

Here are the most common homeopathic remedies used for the common cold:

Polypharmacy: This is a mixed remedy for a generic cold and can be taken without a homeopathic consultation by anyone who wants to take care of general cold symptoms.

Aconite: This is sometimes called a homeopathic vitamin C, because it's useful in the first stages of many common infections, according to Dana Ullman, M.P.H., president of Homeopathic Educational Services in Berkeley, California and author of the *Consumer's Guide to Homeopathy*. Traditionally, aconite is a good remedy to take at the first sign of a cold, according to Dr. Lockie, but it is recommended only during the first 24 hours. It works especially well if you have a cold with sneezing, runny nose, sore throat, and fever. If taken with the first sneeze (especially combined with vitamin C) it is reputed to get rid of some colds overnight.

Anas barbariae (Oscillococcinum): This can ward off colds and flu if taken at the first sign of infection and is the leading cold and flu medicine in Europe, according to Dr. Tom Kruzel, N.D., of Portland, Oregon. It works well because it stimulates the body's own self-defense mechanisms to eliminate the sick or toxic environment in the body.

Belladonna: A deadly poison when taken in normal doses, it is used to treat cold symptoms in the microdoses of homeopathy. Belladonna should be taken when a cold comes on suddenly with high fever, dry skin, sensitive eyes, sore throat, tickly cough, and thirst, according to Dr. Lockie.

Ferrum phosphate 30X: This can help nonspecific cold symptoms if you just don't feel well. It works best when taken at the first sign of a cold.

Oscillococcinum: Use this remedy, recommends Dr. Carrow, every 4 to 6 hours for generalized cold symptoms, together with a tincture of echinacea and goldenseal.

Learn to Manage Your Stress

Mental and emotional stress impairs your immune system's ability to fight off viruses, and doubles your risk of catching a cold. Studies of more than 400 people at Carnegie Mellon University in Pittsburgh found that those who said they had high levels of psychological stress were twice as likely to develop a cold as those with low stress levels. This could be because stress hormones tax the immune system, suggests Sheldon Cohen, Ph.D., professor of psychology at Carnegie Mellon. Relaxation exercises such as meditation can increase the production of immunoglobulin A (IgA), an antibody that helps defend the body against colds. IgA is an immune system protein that acts as the body's first line of defense against colds. The higher the IgA level, the better your chances are of fighting off a cold.

Laugh a Little

As you now know, one measure of a healthy immune system is your IgA level. In one study, researchers found that watching a funny Richard Pryor videotape boosted the viewers' IgA levels significantly, according to Kathleen Dillon, Ph.D., professor of psychology at Western New England College in Springfield, Massachusetts. Those who watched an educational video had no changes in their IgA levels.

Massage Away Your Cold

IgA levels are also affected by massage, according to Boston researchers. Half of a group of elderly research participants lay on massage tables for 10 minutes without massage; the other group had massage. Those who were massaged showed a significant increase in IgA levels.

Think Your Way to Health

According to a Harvard University study, those who use guided imagery, or visualization, are able to boost immune-system elements that fight off colds. The subjects in this study put themselves in a relaxed meditative state and imagined their immune systems attacking cold viruses. They were able to stay cold-free by focusing on this image.

Martin Rossman, M.D., a general practitioner in Mill Valley, California, encourages his patients to practice guided imagery to fight colds. Dr. Rossman believes that a positive attitude can help mobilize your immune system. One of the techniques he suggests is: After entering a relaxed state, imagine an army of tiny maids cleaning up germs in your body with a bucket of disinfectants.

Massage Your Way to Health with Acupressure

Acupressure is based on the same principles as acupuncture (see page 57), in which key points of the body are stimulated to enhance the flow of energy to organs and systems of the body. The difference is that acupressure uses finger pressure to stimulate these points, whereas acupuncture uses thin needles.

If you apply pressure to certain points, you can relieve general cold symptoms, according to Pennsylvania massage therapist Karen Weinrich. For each of these points, apply gentle pressure in a massaging motion for five seconds and then release:

- In hollow of muscle between thumb and index finger.
  Use thumb and one finger to apply gently massaging pressure.

- On inner side of leg, just above upper edge of inner ankle bone, in the hollow between Achilles' tendon and inner edge of tibia

- From the top of the head down to the hollow at the base of the skull

- Across both eyebrows for 1 minute

- The center of the breastbone and a point 3 inches directly below the navel

- One inch below the hollow of each elbow and the hollows on the underside of the knees

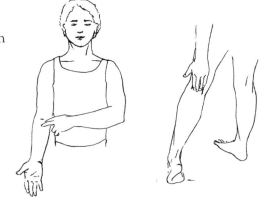

- The big toes and the pads beneath them and the middle toes

- The back of each wrist and the top of each foot where it meets the ankle, using your index and middle fingers

And Then There's Acupuncture

Acupuncture can be a great painless way to treat the symptoms of the cold or flu, according to Dr. Carrow. According to acupuncture experts, the weakened immune system in those with a cold are due to depleted energy, and p-cortisol (a stress adaptation hormone from the adrenal cortex). To rechannel energy levels, acupuncturists use acupuncture meridians related to endocrine function, digestion, lungs, and other organs. When used as a preventive, acupuncture can help those with a long history of chronic cold and flu symptoms remain symptom-free.

Acupuncture not only treats the common cold, it can bring dramatic results with instant relief to the patient, according to Willem Khoe, M.D., acupuncturist with the Department of Modern Acupuncture, Serra Medical Group in Sun Valley, California. While chronic cases may take time to control, acute illnesses can be relieved before you leave the office.

In general, acupuncture is safe and effective if performed by a qualified practitioner. The needles used are so delicate that most people hardly notice them. Needles should be sterilized or disposed of after every use.

After diagnosis, specific needles are placed in some of the more than 1,000 locations on the body—but no more than 10 or 12 needles are used per treatment. The more skillful the acupuncturist, the fewer needles will be needed. The slight pricking sensation you feel when needles are inserted is not painful. The needles are usually as thin as a hair and to protect the patient and acupuncturist, most experts use presterilized, disposable needles. Chinese herbs (teas or pills) also may be given to supplement therapy.

Look for practitioners certified by the National Commission for the Certification of Acupuncturists; in some states, they need to be licensed. Check with your state health department for regulations in your area.

Ice Cube Stimulation

To stimulate the appropriate acupuncture points for a cold, place an ice cube on the bottom of both of your big toes. Keep them in place with an Ace bandage or piece of cloth. (Place your feet in a basin or on plastic to avoid a mess.) Do this morning, noon, and night to help relieve your cold symptoms.

Strengthen Your Immune System with Hydrotherapy

Some experts observe that outbreaks of colds often coincide with dramatic changes in temperature, humidity, and the seasons. Hydrotherapy is another way of strengthening your immune system and helping you to cope with these changes.

When done on a regular basis, contrast hydrotherapy—exposing the body to sudden shifts of hot and cold water—will keep the body and immune system acclimatized. All you need to do is run the last 30 to 60 seconds of a morning shower at a colder temperature.

Try a Sauna

Researchers have found that if you steam yourself in a sauna at least twice a week, you're less likely to catch a cold, according to Dr. Jahre. This could be because the high temperature—just like a fever—may block the cold viruses from reproducing.

Keep Warm and Save Energy

If you get chilled, your body has to use valuable energy to protect you from the cold instead of keeping your immune system focused on your infection. Keep bundled up, advises Keith W. Sehnert, M.D., a physician with Trinity Health Care in Minneapolis, Minnesota, and you'll be able to fight off your cold better.

Make Sure You Rest

If you try to keep on working and pushing yourself when you're sick, you won't have the energy your body needs to fight off the cold. Take a day or two off from work until you feel really well, recommends Dr. Snider. Resting can also help you avoid complications like pneumonia.

If you can't take a day off from work, slow down your activities. If you don't feel well, it's probably going to take you twice as long to accomplish the same tasks anyway. Give your body a break, and relax.

For a good night's sleep, brew a cup of hops or valerian herb teas, which have a tranquilizing effect, according to Dr. Van Ert. Add a teaspoon of honey for a simple sedative.

Stop Smoking!

If you can't stop smoking for good, at least try putting the pack away while you have a cold, advises Samuel Caughron, M.D., a family practitioner specializing in preventive medicine in Charlottesville, Virginia. Smoking not only aggravates a sore throat, it can interfere with the infection-fighting cilia that sweep bacteria out of your lungs and throat.

If You Have Recurrent Colds...

Remember that if you have recurrent colds, you should get a complete medical check-up to rule out common undetected causes of immune problems, such as hypothyroidism, thyroiditis, systemic candidiasis, food allergies, chronic sinusitis, and a weakened adrenal gland.

Exercise to Boost Your Immune System

People who regularly exercise suffer only half as many days with cold symptoms compared with couch potatoes. But extremely strenuous exercise weakens the immune system, and increases your risk of getting a cold. Aim for a happy medium: exercise several times a week —not every day. The amount and type of exercise you try depends on how old you are, your condition, and your general health. Young and strong athletes can choose from a wide range of exercises. But if you're not in such good shape, or you're older or ill, choose a less demanding form. No matter what your condition, don't exercise to the point of exhaustion.

Some researchers believe a daily walk can help get your natural killer cells moving. A daily 45-minute walk can help speed up recovery from colds, according to studies conducted by David Nieman, Ph.D., a health researcher at Appalachian State University in Boone, North Carolina. You know the pace is right if you can comfortably talk while you're walking.

Keith W. Sehnert, M.D., a physician with Trinity Health Care in Minneapolis, Minnesota, also recommends walking to boost your immune system. Another good gentle exercise, says Dr. Sehnert, is jumping on a rebounder for 15 minutes.

In the Next Chapter

If a sore throat is bothering you, read on to the next chapter where you'll find lots of natural ways to get rid of the sore, scratchy, irritated throat that so often accompanies the common cold.

CHAPTER ✦ FOUR

27 All-Natural
Sore Throat Remedies

NE OF THE MOST common symptoms of a cold is a scratchy, sore, inflamed throat. Your throat feels swollen and tender, and it hurts when you swallow. While most sore throats run their course in a few days or weeks, the pain can be severe while they last. Most sore throats are caused by a cold virus, and develop gradually over a period of days. If there is a fever, it's not usually more than 101 degrees F.

A bacterial throat infection, on the other hand (caused either by the streptococcus or staphylococcus bacteria), usually comes on fast; lymph glands are often tender, and a headache develops. Fever is usually 102 degrees F or more, and your throat may be very red, with white or yellow spots. You'll need a throat culture to tell the difference between a sore throat caused by bacteria and one caused by a cold virus. Still, only about 15 percent of all sore throats are caused by bacteria.

If you're wondering if that scractchy throat is just a cold symptom or something caused by bacteria that would require treatment with antibiotics, there are a couple of ways to help you decide. It's probably a bacterial infection if you have:

- lingering voice problems
- swallowing problems
- sore throat that lasts more than three days

See your doctor if you think you have a sore throat caused by a bacterial infection. If you don't have the above symptoms, odds are your sore throat is the result of one of the many cold viruses. In that case, the natural remedies in this chapter will help ease the pain.

Use Zinc to Relieve Your Pain

Long suspected to be a solid treatment for colds, zinc lozenges can be a real help for a sore throat, according to Michelle Moore, M.D., of Keene, New Hampshire. A recent study found that indeed, those who used zinc lozenges got over their sore throat and other cold symptoms three days faster than those who didn't. Some people, however, were not pleased with the taste of the zinc. For that reason, scientists have developed a variety of flavored zinc lozenges that can now be found in health food stores.

For best results, dissolve one zinc gluconate lozenge by mouth every 2 hours until the pain is gone. Don't use more than 12 in 24 hours, and not for longer than one week. Because the taste of unflavored zinc is notoriously bad, if you're not taking a flavored lozenge, try sucking a peppermint candy at the same time to mask the unpleasant taste.

The recommended daily intake for prevention is 15 mg., and experts recommend taking six lozenges each containing 11.5 mg. per day for a total of 69 mg if you have a cold. Don't overuse, however; over a long period of time, this much zinc could interfere with the absorption of copper, according to Dr. Trevor Delves, consultant biochemist at England's Southhampton University NHS Trust.

It may be necessary to eat a cracker before taking the zinc if zinc makes you feel a little sick to your stomach, according to Donald J. Carrow, M.D., of Clearwater, Florida.

Suck On Hard Candies and Lozenges

Sucking butterscotch candy throughout the day can ease the pain of a sore throat and is the favorite personal remedy of Steven J. Pearl-man, M.D., associate director of the Department of Otolaryngology at the St. Luke's/Roosevelt Hospital Center in New York City. The candy doesn't kill germs, but it does boost the production of saliva and can soothe a painful throat.

Dr. Pearlman notes that many other types of nonprescription lozenges (some of which contain a mild anesthetic) can provide temporary pain relief as well.

Menthol Can Cool Your Throat

Anything containing menthol — such as hard lozenges or candies — can ease a burning sore throat, according to Ron Eccles, M.D., director of the Common Cold Centre, School of Molecular and Medical Biosciences, University of Wales, Cardiff, Wales. Mint tea can also help ease the pain of a sore throat because the oil in mint is menthol. Try this recipe:

Mint Tea

1 handful or bunch of fresh mint leaves, or 2 teaspoons dried mint leaves
1 cup boiling water

Steep leaves for 10 minutes in boiling water. Drink up to 3 cups a day.

Gargle Your Pain Away

Gargling can temporarily ease the pain of a sore throat, shrink swollen tissue, break up congestion, and help flush out bacteria. It's a great remedy for a sore throat, according to Alan Cohen, M.D., medical director of Harmony Health Care in Milford, Connecticut. You'll get the best results from gargling if you have the kind of sore throat that hurts when you swallow. This indicates the sore tissue is high enough in the throat for the gargle solution to reach it.

Avoid gargling with prepared mouthwashes. Instead, "there's nothing much better than gargling with salt water," says Jack Gwaltney, M.D., chief of epidemiology and virology at the University of Virginia School of Medicine. For a good salt water gargle, mix 1 teaspoon of salt into 8 ounces of warm water and gargle with it every 20 to 30 minutes, according to Annette Stoesser, M.D., of Roswell, New Mexico.

Other experts like the bubbling action of hydrogen peroxide, which can soothe the throat by oxygenating your tissues, according to otolaryngologist Charles Kimmelman, M.D., physician at Manhattan Eye, Ear, and Throat Hospital in New York City. For a good hydrogen peroxide gargle, mix a 3 percent solution with water, four times a day. Spit the mix out immediately after gargling.

Herbalists recommend that you ease a painful sore throat with any of the following mixtures:

HALF-AND-HALF GARGLE

Combine equal portions of water with one of the following:
aloe vera gel
apple cider vinegar
lemon juice
pekoe tea

BREWER'S YEAST AND HONEY GARGLE

Combine:
¼ cup brewer's yeast
1 tablespoon honey
1 cup water

Honey and Water Gargle

Combine:
¼ cup honey
¼ cup cider vinegar
¼ cup water

Currant Gargle

Simmer for 10 minutes:
1 tablespoon dried currants
1 cup water

Add:
½ teaspoon cinnamon
Cover, let stand for 30 minutes, and then strain.

Pomegranate Gargle

Boil until reduced to 2 cups:
2 tablespoons dried grated pomegranate rind
3 cups water

Cool, then strain.

Chamomile Tea Gargle

Steep:
1 teaspoon dried chamomile flowers
1 cup hot water

Strain. Cool to lukewarm, and gargle as needed.

Cayenne Pepper Gargle

Steep in 1 cup boiling water:
2 teaspoons cayenne pepper
2 teaspoons dried sage

Then stir in:
2 teaspoons honey
2 teaspoons salt
2 teaspoons vinegar

Strain.

Baking Soda Gargle

Combine:
¼ to ½ teaspoon salt
¼ to ½ teaspoon baking soda
½ cup warm water

Vinegar Gargle

Combine:
1 tablespoon cider vinegar
8 ounces water
(This solution can be irritating to some; if so, discontinue.)

Goldenseal Gargle

Another good way to gargle is to make an infusion with 1 teaspoon goldenseal and 1 cup warm water, according to Dr. Moore. The goldenseal and water can be soothing and healing to inflamed throat tissues.

◆❖◆ CAUTION: Goldenseal should not be used by pregnant women.

Try a Beverage with Cayenne Pepper

In addition to making a good gargle, herbalists recommend a beverage of cayenne pepper and ginger ale to ease sore throat pain. Cayenne also tastes good added to warm lemon juice and honey, according to Dr. Moore. The cayenne will boost the production of saliva, which can restore the acid-base balance in the throat.

Mix Up a Hot Sauce Cocktail

Many physicians recommend hot spicy flavors to ease the pain of a sore throat. Here's a recipe for a hot sauce cocktail from Dr. Carrow:

small glass of vegetable juice
hot cocktail sauce (as much as you can stand)

Add the sauce to the vegetable juice. Gargle several times with the mixture, allowing it to slowly drain down your throat. This will clear up most sore throats, Dr. Carrow says. It is also a great preventive if used daily.

Drink Lots of Liquids

One of the problems of a sore throat is that the tissues are too dry; this is one reason why doctors are always telling you to drink plenty of fluids when you get sick. Drinking lots of beverages will help hydrate those sore, dried-out throat tissues, according to Dr. Eccles and James Schuler, M.D., of Smith River, California. Anything tasty that stimulates salivation and respiratory tract secretions will do well, recommends Dr. Eccles. Even if you're not feeling thirsty, warns Dr. Schuler, make sure you drink plenty of fluids, including juices, throughout the day.

Avoid drinking cold liquids, which can increase congestion, and milk, which can produce more mucus. Since caffeinated beverages act as diuretics, robbing your body of fluid, it's best not to drink these either. Cold viruses multiply best at temperatures slightly below normal body temperature, so drinking hot soup or liquid can ease a sore throat by raising your body temperature, thereby diminishing viral reproduction.

Since acidic beverages can thin the mucus lining of the throat, they are a good choice when you have a cold, according to Dr. Eccles. Try drinking warm orange, lemon, or tomato juice, or warm lemonade made with honey and fresh lemons. Hot tasty soups are another good choice. A mixture of 1 tablespoon of cider vinegar or apple cider, honey, and a glass of warm water is another good recipe, according to Dr. Stoesser. While these tart beverages work well because they are acidic, for the same reason they also can be irritating to sensitive throat tissue. If citrus-based liquids bother your throat, try sipping any honey- sweetened tea, such as bayberry root bark, catnip, ginger, or hyssop.

Or mix 1 tablespoon pure horseradish with 1 teaspoon each of honey and ground cloves into a cup of warm water. Sip slowly and keep stirring to prevent the horseradish from sinking to the bottom of the glass. This beverage may also be used as a gargle.

Another favorite remedy from Dr. Moore is:

Lemon Juice Hot Drink

½ cup warm fresh lemon juice
honey to taste
pinch of cayenne pepper

Mix all 3 ingredients together; drink often to ease the pain.

Use Salt Spray to Stay Hydrated

To keep your throat moist, use a saline nasal spray. You can find these sprays marketed under several different brand names at your local drug store. The salty spray first helps to moisten your nasal passages; then, it drips down the back of your throat to rehydrate parched tissues, according to Dr. Surow. These sprays are not habit-forming and won't harm your nose.

Humidify

Many researchers believe that breathing a cool mist can help ease the pain of a sore throat, according to Dr. Moore. This is because dry air interferes with the effectiveness of the nasal cilia, those long hairlike fingers that sweep the incoming air clear of viruses and bacteria. Using a humidifier or a cool-mist vaporizer also can help keep the lining of the throat moist.

If you use a cool-air vaporizer, it's important to keep it clean; improperly-maintained machines can emit dust mites and mold spores into the air, and ultrasonic humidifiers can coat furniture with a film that can trigger allergies and sore throats.

For a really bad sore throat, you can supplement your humidifier with steam inhalations. Let hot water run into the bathroom sink until the room gets steamy; then place a towel over your head and lean over the basin, inhaling deeply through the mouth and nose for 5 to 10 minutes. Try inhaling the steam several times a day to soothe irritation. For added benefit, add a teaspoon of tincture of benzoin (or menthol or eucalyptus oil) to the hot water.

Keep Your Mouth Closed

To prevent dry air from irritating an already-inflamed throat, it will help to keep your mouth closed while breathing.

A recurrent sore throat may be traced to sleeping with your mouth open or your head too low. To prevent this, tilt your bed frame so your head is about five inches higher than your feet. (Don't just add pillows; this adds pressure to the esophagus and can worsen the condition.)

"Coat" Your Sore Throat with Petroleum Jelly

A pinch of petroleum jelly put on your lower teeth and smashed with the tongue and then swallowed can ease the pain of a sore throat, according to David Darbo, M.D., of Indianapolis, Indiana.

Apply a Compress or Poultice

Some experts, including Dr. Schuler, swear by the use of a hot compress. Apply a comfortably hot pack against the front of your throat for about 15 minutes. Repeat up to seven times a day. Dr. Schuler also recommends applying a warm compress to your throat and then sleeping with a muffler wrapped around your throat to ease the pain.

Alternatively, you can apply a warm chamomile poultice directly to the outside of the throat. To prepare:

CHAMOMILE POULTICE

Mix 1 tablespoon dried chamomile flowers to 1 or 2 cups of boiling water. Steep for five minutes, and then strain. Dip a clean cloth in the mixture and then apply to the throat until the cloth loses heat. Repeat as often as necessary.

Acupressure or Massage for Your Sore Throat

More than 5,000 years ago, Chinese healers noticed that when you press and massage certain parts of the body you can relieve certain ailments. Experts believe today that this works due to the release of "energy blocks" in the meridians (healing lines) around the body. (See Chapter 3, page 55.) This technique is called acupressure, and it uses the pressure of hands and fingers to affect the health of the body by improving circulation and stimulating the movement of blood and lymph from tissues.

There are several different areas of the body that can be manipulated to ease sore throats. Here are three different techniques recommended by certified massage therapists:

ACUPRESSURE TECHNIQUE I

- First, apply gentle pressure in a circular massaging motion for 5 seconds on the lower part of each thumb and the web that attaches it to the hand, and then release.

- Then press the bottom of each thumbnail on the side closest to the index finger. With the right thumbnail, press the bottom outside corner of the left thumbnail for 7 seconds. Release and repeat 3 times. Then go through the whole procedure again with the right thumbnail.

ACUPRESSURE TECHNIQUE II

- Massage each big toe and the web between it and the next toe.

ACUPRESSURE TECHNIQUE III

- Push down on the top margin of the breastbone for 10 seconds. Release for 10 seconds. Repeat 3 times.

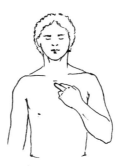

Sip Syrups to Soothe Your Throat

The soothing taste and consistency of a spoonful of sugar- or honey-based syrups can ease many a sore throat. Here are several different recipes for old-time favorites:

- Combine equal amounts of brown sugar and brandy.
- Blend honey and bee pollen in equal amounts.
- Combine equal parts of egg white, honey, and lemon juice.
- Mix ¼ cup hot lemon juice, ½ cup honey, and 1 tablespoon glycerin.
- Steep peeled garlic cloves in honey for several days, then strain and sip syrup.

Numb Your Throat with Cloves

To numb the pain of a sore throat, suck on a whole clove. In the days before modern anesthesia, dentists used clove oil as a local anesthetic. It may taste bitter, but it should work in minutes. Some experts recommend chewing whole cloves, but no more than four a day. Make sure you spit out the cloves after chewing; if you swallow them, they can upset your stomach.

◆◆CAUTION: Do not use clove oil for a sore throat, since swallowing clove oil can cause stomach problems.

Use Garlic, Nature's Antibiotic and Antiseptic

Considered by herbal experts to be one of the best natural antiseptics and antibiotics available, garlic is a popular choice for restoring overall health. It also can be used to ease a sore throat. To try this remedy, take two 15-grain garlic-oil capsules with each meal. The advantage of using garlic pills or capsules rather than raw garlic is that you avoid the powerful smell on your breath. Purists, however, insist on nothing but the real thing; they find relief by holding a clove of garlic in the mouth (followed by the use of breath mints).

Try Licorice Root for Easing Throat Inflammation

True licorice—not the candy, but the root of the plant—can ease the pain of a sore throat, according to physician Richard Kunin, M.D., of San Francisco, California. Products made from the roots and rhizome of European licorice (*Glycyyrrhiza glabra*) or other related members of the licorice species—all members of the pea family—are very effective for soothing sore, inflamed tissue. Available in health food stores as a powder or candy, the root owes its sweetness and healing power to glycyrrhetinic acid, a compound 50 times sweeter than sugar. It is used widely in Europe in sore-throat formulas, but because of its overpowering sweetness, true licorice is not often used in commercial American candies.

You can find licorice in natural food stores in capsules, lozenges, powders, concentrated drops, tinctures, and extracts. Chewable tablets and other licorice products for extended use often contain only two percent or less of the active ingredient glycyrrhizic acid. These products—called "deglycyrrhizinated licorice" or DGL—cause fewer side effects (see warning below) and are much safer for long-term use. An average dose of DGL is about 200 mg. To use, sprinkle a pinch of the powdered herb into hot water or tea. Use for about a week.

❖❖ CAUTION: Don't use more than a half ounce (about 3 teaspoons) of the powder daily over several weeks. Larger or repeated doses of licorice extracts containing glycyrrhizin may cause headaches, lethargy, water retention, high blood pressure, and excess excretion of potassium. Because of these side effects, avoid using licorice if you are pregnant or you have diabetes, glaucoma, high blood pressure, heart disease, or stroke.

Use Marsh Mallow for Soothing Throat Irritation

Real marsh mallow is an herb with a long root found growing in marshes that can soothe irritation in the throat, according to the late

Heinz Rosler, Ph.D., formerly of the department of medicinal chemistry at the University of Maryland School of Pharmacy in Baltimore. It is no longer an ingredient in puffy white marshmallows that float in your morning cocoa. However, in the 1800s doctors extracted the juice from the plant's roots and cooked it with egg whites and sugar, whipping it into a meringue that, once hardened, was used as a medicinal candy to soothe a child's sore throat.

While not widely available in the United States, some health food stores carry marsh mallow tea or crushed marsh mallow root. The flowers, roots, and leaves of the plant all contain a thick, gooey substance called mucilage that swells and becomes slippery as it absorbs water.

To make a marsh mallow tea, boil for 10 to 15 minutes:
½ to 1 teaspoon crushed root
1 cup water

Try Mullein, a Soothing Herbal Remedy

This herbal remedy for sore throats also contains mucilage, which accounts for its soothing effect on a painful throat. Mullein can be taken as a tincture in doses of ½ to 1 teaspoon up to three times a day.

As a tea, use 1 to 2 teaspoons dried leaves per cup; allow to steep for 10 minutes. You can drink up to three cups per day. Because of its bitter taste, you may want to add sugar or honey for sweetness.

The U.S. Food and Drug Administration includes mullein on its list of GRAS herbs (herbs that are "generally recognized as safe"). While the seeds of the plant are toxic, there have been no reports of poisoning with leaves, flowers, or roots. However, mullein has tannins, which have been suspected as having both cancer-causing and cancer-fighting properties. For this reason, to be safe, herbalists suggest that no one with a history of cancer take mullein internally.

Grow Your Own Marsh Mallow

The marsh mallow plant can be found in boggy, damp areas and along streams. The 5-foot-tall perennial has a long taproot whose stems die back each autumn. The plant produces pink or white flowers in summer.

To grow your own marsh mallow, plant in moist soil in areas that receive full sun. The plant can be propagated from seeds, cuttings, or root division in autumn. Seeds can be obtained from most mail order herb farms. (See Appendix B.)

The roots should be harvested only from plants more than two years old. When the top growth has died back in fall, dig up the mature roots and wash, peel, and dry them whole or in slices.

Drink Sage Tea, a Natural Antiseptic

Because of its antiseptic qualities, sage tea can take the sting out of a sore throat, according to herb expert Varro Tyler, Ph.D, professor at Purdue University. To make sage tea, pour a cup of boiling water over 1 to 2 teaspoons of dried leaves and steep for 10 minutes.

Use Slippery Elm to Ease Your Pain

Slippery elm, which is derived from the inner bark of the elm tree, can be a soothing remedy for a sore throat, according to Dr. Moore.

Slippery elm has been reviewed by the FDA as safe and effective for treating sore throats.

Health food stores carry slippery elm lozenges, and a powder for tea. To make the tea, add 1 teaspoon of slippery elm powder to 1 cup of hot water and an equal amount of milk; sweeten with sugar. Health food stores also carry ready-made slippery elm tea; try combining this with ¼ teaspoon goldenseal and an equal amount of milk.

Take Yin Chiao Chieh Tu Pien Tablets at the First Sign of a Sore Throat

This traditional Chinese formula, sold as tablets in health food stores, contains honeysuckle and forsythia. But you should use more than the dosage given on the box, according to Linda Wright, M.D., of Boulder, Colorado. At the first sign of a sore throat, take 3 to 5 tablets of Yin Chiao every two to three hours until symptoms subside. The tablets can help keep severe sore throat symptoms from developing.

Try Nutrient-Rich Elderberry

This popular herb used for a wide variety of ills is most commonly used to treat a sore throat caused by the common cold. Elderberry is made from the flowers and dark purple berries of the black or common elder tree, a small European tree. It can be bought in health food stores as a lozenge, throat spray, tincture, syrup, or liquid extract. Follow dosage directions found on the label.

The berries of the tree contain vitamin C, flavonoids, tannins, and other plant nutrients, some of which may bind to the virus and prevent it from attacking cells, according to research. Elderberry flowers contain flavonoids, mucilage, tannins, and other healing compounds.

While substances made from the berry or flowers of the elderberry can be taken internally, avoid ingesting elderberry products made from the bark or leaves.

Try Osha, a Native American Throat Remedy

Also known as Porter's lovage, this herb belongs to the carrot family and has been used for hundreds of years by Native Americans to treat sore throats. Osha helps ease painful throats by keeping mucus wet and fluid, according to New Mexico herbalist Daniel Gagnon, executive director of the Botanical Research and Education Institute. The part of the herb used for medicine is the root. You can take 30 drops of the liquid extract, or one capsule every 3 to 4 hours, up to 5 times a day.

◆⋅◆CAUTION: Do not use osha during pregnancy.

Vitamins A, C, and E

Originally known as the "anti-infective vitamin, vitamin A plays an essential role in maintaining the integrity of the lining of the respiratory tract..." according to Michael Murray, N.D. and Joseph Pizzorno, N.D., in *An Encyclopedia of Natural Medicine.*

Gargling with 500 mg. of powdered vitamin C in a glass of water, together with a 250 mg. vitamin C tablet each hour, can ease a sore throat very quickly. In addition, to aid healing of the sore throat and to strengthen the immune system, try: 75,000 IU of beta carotene (provitamin A) daily for one week, followed by 50,000 IU for one week, followed by 25,000 IU daily until the pain subsides. Or try 25,000 IU of vitamin A per day until your throat feels better.

In addition, Dr. Kunin recommends dissolving 100 IU vitamin E capsules (preferably synthetic d-alpha tocopherol acetate) in your mouth once a day to ease sore throat pain.

In the Next Chapter

For more information on treating a fever the natural way, read on to the next chapter, where experts offer a host of effective home remedies.

15 Ways to Reduce
Fever Naturally

A FEVER IS NOT AN ILLNESS — it's the way your body tries to fight infection. Since most disease-causing organisms can't reproduce at high temperatures, cranking up your internal temperature helps your body fight a cold.

For this reason, a fever really shouldn't be suppressed, according to Tom Kruzel, N.D., in private practice in Portland, Oregon. Most people run for the bottle of aspirin or acetaminophen as soon as the thermometer inches above 99 degrees F. But as long as it doesn't go too high, it's best to leave a fever alone and let your body work to make you better.

Although a body temperature of 98.6 degrees F is considered normal, few people actually maintain that exact temperature, even when they are completely healthy. Children also tend to have higher temperatures than adults, and more variations throughout the day. Generally, a temperature range between 99 degrees to 100 degrees F could be considered a fever, according to Donald Vickery, M.D., assistant clinical professor at Georgetown University School of Medicine. Anything over 100 degrees F is definitely a fever.

It's generally safe to let an adult's body temperature rise untreated until it gets to about 103 degrees F; after that, a fever can become more serious.

To bring down a fever, there are a number of effective natural remedies you can try.

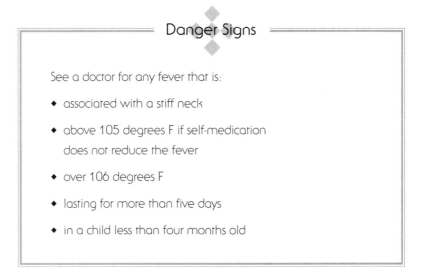

Danger Signs

See a doctor for any fever that is:

- associated with a stiff neck

- above 105 degrees F if self-medication does not reduce the fever

- over 106 degrees F

- lasting for more than five days

- in a child less than four months old

Drink Liquids to Stay Hydrated

When you're hot, your body perspires to cool itself down, but if you perspire *too much* (as you can with a high fever), you can become dehydrated and your body stops sweating to save on water. This makes it harder to cope with fever. To make sure your body stays hydrated, try drinking as much of any of these beverages as you can for as long as your fever lasts:

WATER

Water is still the very best clear liquid you can drink to help your body rehydrate itself and cope with fever. Sip cool water throughout the day—8 glasses at least. If so much water bothers your stomach, try alternating with sips of ginger ale.

Fruit or vegetable juices

Beet and carrot juice are filled with vitamins and minerals and make an excellent choice for a hydrating drink, according to Eleonore Blaurock-Busch, Ph.D., president and director of Trace Minerals International in Boulder, Colorado. Drink as much as you can during the day.

Thyme/linden/chamomile tea

Steep 1 teaspoon equal parts of these herbs in 1 cup of boiling water for 5 minutes; strain and drink warm several times a day. The chamomile will reduce inflammation, the thyme has antiseptic properties, and linden flowers promote sweating.

Linden flower tea

Linden tea alone is helpful if you need to bring down a fever, according to Dr. Blaurock-Busch. Use 1 tablespoon of flowers in 1 cup of boiling water, and drink hot as often as necessary.

Willow bark tea

Willow bark is the favored tea used by Native Americans to break fevers. Rich in salicylates (aspirin-related compounds), the tea can be brewed and drunk in small doses to bring down a fever, once or twice a day.

Lemon balm tea

Steep dried lemon balm leaves in hot water, add honey and lemon. Drink 2 or 3 cups per day while the fever lasts.

LEMON WATER

Try combining the juice of a lemon, 1 pint of water, and 1 teaspoon of cream of tartar; sweeten to taste. Drink freely while the fever lasts.

HOT LEMON AND HONEY

Combine equal portions of lemon and honey, and heat through; drink as often as necessary until the fever breaks.

ICE

High fevers may be associated with nausea; if you don't think you can drink *anything,* try sucking on ice or frozen fruit juice as often as you wish while the fever lasts.

Drink Pepper to Break Your Fever

When you drink or eat spicy-hot chili peppers, that spicy flavor is stimulating your circulation and boosting your ability to sweat, according to medical experts. Because of this sweat-producing property, cayenne pepper and other related chili peppers are sometimes used to break a fever.

The important ingredient here is capsaicin, the active ingredient in many over-the-counter drug preparations used primarily for skin conditions and arthritis. In addition to the real vegetable, you can buy cayenne as a capsule, concentrated drop, or tincture—all of which are taken internally. Most popular products contain between 5 to 10 percent capsaicin, and an average dose of an 8 percent oral capsaicin product, according to herbalists, is about 100 mg.

❖❖❖CAUTION: If you're handling chili peppers, remember that they can cause serious tissue irritation. Wash your hands well after handling peppers or the capsaicin cream, and avoid touching mucous membranes, your eyes, or open wounds. If you use too much, you can inflame the lining of your stomach and harm your kidneys. If you use packaged products, follow package directions carefully and don't use more than the recommended dose.

Herbalists have created a variety of drinks that include cayenne pepper. Here's a good one:

PEPPER AND HONEY DRINK

Boil 4 cups of water with ½ teaspoon cayenne pepper. As you're ready to drink a cup, heat the pepper water with 1 teaspoon honey and ¼ cup orange juice. Drink slowly.

Feed a Cold, Feed a Fever

That old myth about feeding a cold and starving a fever is just plain wrong, according to health experts. Since your body burns energy more quickly when you have a fever, you need more calories. The problem, however, is that a fever will usually kill your appetite. To fuel your body without aggravating your lack of appetite, try simple, basic foods. Some dietary winners for folks with fevers are:

◆ bananas
◆ plain custards
◆ simple soups (especially chicken-based)
◆ gelatin desserts (such as Jello)
◆ applesauce
◆ bouillon

Use Compresses to Reduce Your Temperature

Hot, moist compresses can help reduce the body's temperature if it is less than 103 degrees F by forcing the body to perspire more as a way to cool itself. If the compresses make you feel too uncomfortable, remove them and replace with cool compresses on forehead, wrist, and calves. Keep the rest of the body covered.

Fevers over 103 degrees F can be brought down by applying cool compresses; they should be changed as they warm to body temperature. Continue until the fever breaks. You can also try sandwiching your body between cool wet towels, changing them every 15 minutes.

Take Sponge Baths

A tepid sponge bath can help cut a high fever because the air moving over the damp skin has a cooling effect on the body, according to James Schuler, M.D., of Smith River, California. Concentrate on areas that are hottest (usually the armpits and groin). Wring out a sponge in tepid water, wipe one section at a time, keeping the rest of the body covered. You don't need to dry the area with towels because body heat will evaporate the moisture.

Do not use alcohol because its faster evaporation rate may be uncomfortable to someone with a fever. There is also the danger of absorbing the alcohol through the skin or inhaling the vapor, especially in children.

For Chills, Take a Warm Bath and Cover Up

If your high fever is causing chills, you may feel better by taking a warm tub bath, according to Dr. Schuler. M.D. Just be sure not to get too chilled when you get out of the warm water. A room-temperature bath is best for children suffering from chills, according to Leonard Banco, M.D., associate professor of pediatrics at the University of Connecticut medical school. Children don't have a well-developed ability to regulate body temperature, so it's best to keep the water lukewarm rather than too hot.

When you get out of the bath, towel off thoroughly, put on some warm bedclothes and pile on the quilts and comforters until you're comfortable. If all those covers eventually make you feel too hot, take off extra covers. If you've got so many covers that you start to sweat, you'll need to expose your skin to the air so your body heat can dissipate along with your sweat. This is particularly important with feverish infants, who can't take their clothes on and off and who may have problems kicking off covers. Overdressing a child or piling on too many covers may actually cause or worsen a fever.

Work Up a Sweat

To increase metabolism and speed elimination of the cold virus, some health practitioners recommend "sweating therapy." Drink 2 cups of hot ginger lemonade (see page 90), get in bed, cover up with several blankets, and sweat (but not to the point of exhaustion). Follow this with a cool water sponge bath, change the sheets, and get back into bed.

Others recommend keeping the lower part of your body very warm, such as with a heating pad or hot water bottle on your feet.

In any case, staying warm will help you feel more comfortable, especially if you have a fever, according to Donald Girard, M.D., head of the division of general internal medicine at Oregon Health Sciences University in Portland.

Turn Down the Heat

Don't keep the thermostat cranked up if you've got a fever. Instead, allow fresh air in but don't create a draft, according to Dr. Blaurock-Busch. Dr. Benjamin Spock has long recommended a cool bedroom temperature (about 65 degrees F) for optimum health.

Get Some Rest

You probably won't be feeling well enough to run around the block if you have a fever, but be sure to get plenty of rest. Exercising or

How to Use a Thermometer

USING A GLASS/MERCURY ORAL THERMOMETER

Wait at least 30 minutes after eating, drinking, or smoking before taking an oral temperature.

◆ Hold thermometer by top end (not bulb) and shake with a quick snap of the wrist until mercury drops below 96 degrees F.

◆ Hold thermometer under the tongue in a pocket on either side of the mouth, not right up front. (The pockets are closer to blood vessels that reflect the body's core temperature.)

◆ Hold the thermometer with your lips (not teeth). Breathe through your nose.

◆ Leave in place for at least 3 minutes (some say 5 to 7 minutes).

USING A RECTAL THERMOMETER

Use a rectal thermometer in children under age 5. Rectal thermometers have a short, round bulb. Be aware that rectal temperature is usually 1 degree warmer than oral temperature.

◆ Place child (stomach down) on your lap and hold one hand on buttocks.

- Lubricate end of thermometer with petroleum jelly; carefully insert about 1 inch—NEVER USE FORCE.

- Remove when mercury stops rising (between 1 and 2 minutes).

- If the thermometer breaks in the rectum, don't panic. Mercury is not poisonous and usually there will be only mild scratches of the lining of the rectum. Call your doctor if you can't find all the pieces of glass.

- Wash thermometer in cool, soapy water. Never use hot water, and never store near heat.

USING A DIGITAL IN-THE-EAR THERMOMETER

Before choosing this type of thermometer, be aware that some physicians believe that a digital thermometer is not as accurate as a glass/mercury instrument.

- Use thermometer according to directions on the package.

- After use, wash the tip with soap and lukewarm water or rubbing alcohol.

- Don't immerse the thermometer or splash water on the readout.

- Change the batteries every two years.

physically exerting yourself when you have a fever will only make matters worse. Those who don't get enough rest during a cold and fever will take longer to recover. You will also expose others to infection if you're out and about.

Fry Up Some Onions

Herbalists often mention onions as a well-known folk remedy for fevers, although no one seems to know why they are supposed to work. Try frying several chopped onions and placing in a small paper bag. Cover your chest with a towel and place the bag on the towel.

Take Cold-Fighting Echinacea

This popular cold-fighting herb and extract of the purple coneflower is an effective antiviral and immune stimulant. It's particularly useful against fever because it stimulates sweating. More than 100 studies have been published on this herbal immune stimulant. "Research... done mostly in Germany has confirmed its antiviral, antibacterial, and immune-enhancing properties," according to well-known physician and best-selling author Andrew Weil, M.D., in *Natural Health, Natural Medicine*.

It may be taken every 2 hours in either capsule, powder, or tincture form. For long-term use, take 3 times a day for 6 to 8 weeks; then discontinue for 2 to 4 weeks. (Echinacea becomes less effective when taken for more than eight weeks at a time.)

Try Feverfew

The leaves and small white flowers of the bushy perennial feverfew have traditionally been used to reduce fever. Sold dried in capsules, concentrated drops, tinctures, or extracts, the newest products have standardized amounts (between 0.1 and 0.2 percent) of a chemical called parthenolide. Herbalists often prescribe an average daily dose of 125 mg. of feverfew (at 0.2 percent parthenolide).

Be aware that studies over the past decade have found that some commercial feverfew products actually contain none of the active compound (parthenolide); keeping feverfew in storage also results in a decrease in the levels of parthenolide. For this reason, it is important to use high-quality extracts of this herb; in addition, don't keep old feverfew products on your shelf.

There are few side effects of this herb. Eating the fresh leaves, however, may cause lip and tongue swelling.

Use Fever-Reducing Elderberry

Many products derived from the elderberry tree's yellow flowers and purple berries can be used to help reduce a fever, according to herbalist experts. It works to reduce fever by inducing sweating in anyone who ingests its flowers or berries. You can find elderberry in your local health food store as a tincture, liquid extract, a lozenge, syrup, extract capsule, or throat spray.

You can also drink tea made from the berries and flowers of the black elder.

Drink Ginger to Cut Your Fever

The underground rhizome of the tropical plant Zingiber officinale has been used since ancient times as both a medicine and flavoring. Today, herbalists recommend ginger as a way to reduce fever in some people. It can be bought in a wide variety of ways, including as a fresh or dried root, tablets, capsules, tinctures, syrups, extracts, and teas. No matter which product you buy, follow directions found on the label. Even relatively large doses of ginger (up to several grams) have not been reported to cause toxicity or side effects. (The essential oil of ginger, however, should not be taken internally.)

A hot drink made with ginger can break a high fever. Try this popular remedy:

Hot Ginger Lemonade

2 inch piece of gingerroot

2 cups boiling water

2 tablespoons lemon juice

1 tablespoon honey

pinch cayenne pepper

Grate the gingerroot into the boiling water, and simmer in a covered pot for 5 minutes. Add lemon juice, honey, and cayenne pepper.

In the Next Chapter

The next chapter provides lots of home remedies for relieving that achy feeling or a congestion headache that often accompanies a cold.

CHAPTER SIX

14 Natural Ways to Stop
Headaches and Body Aches

N UPPER RESPIRATORY TRACT infection (a head cold) can bring on a headache so strong it feels as if the top of your skull will explode. It's usually the result of sinus and nasal congestion; the virus irritates mucous membranes in the nose and sinuses, making them swell and closing off the sinus' tiny openings into the nose. The result is a painful vacuum. If the openings stay closed for too long, the sinuses can fill up with fluid and become infected.

Along with headaches, colds also can bring on general aches caused by muscle pain when the virus itself infects the muscle tissue. As the virus spreads throughout the muscles, it can cause inflammation and pain. This is particularly common with influenza virus type B.

Put a Cold Compress—
or Bag of Frozen Veggies—on Your Head

For a painful headache, try a cold compress on your forehead. The cold will constrict blood vessels in your head, reducing the pain.

One of the fastest ways to ease a headache is to put ice on the area, according to Fred Sheftell, M.D., director of the New England Center for Headaches in Stamford, Connecticut, and coauthor of *Headache Relief*. An ice pack or a bag of frozen vegetables in a towel on the forehead or top of the head together with a warm foot bath is the remedy recommended by James Schuler, M.D., of Smith River, California.

Raise Your Head While You Sleep

One of the reasons many people with colds wake up with a headache is because they were lying flat all night, allowing their sinuses to fill with fluid. In order to help keep your sinuses draining all night and cut down the risk of a headache, go to sleep on your back with your head raised on two to three pillows.

Raising the upper half of your body this way also cuts down on chest congestion and can ease a cough that may accompany your cold.

For a Sinus Headache, Eat a Jalapeno Pepper

As soon as you notice the beginnings of a headache linked to stuffy sinuses, eat a jalapeno pepper. Within minutes, your sinuses will start to drain and the headache will subside. Spicy foods loosen up mucus secretions and boost blood flow to the sinuses.

Try Horseradish As a Decongestant

Horseradish is a member of the mustard family, and it contains pungent aromatic oils that can act as a potent decongestant, which will ease your headache pain. Always use fresh grated horseradish; bottled horseradish does not have the same effect. (Even fresh grated horseradish quickly loses its decongestant properties.)

For an effective horseradish cure:

Grate 1 teaspoon of fresh horseradish, and mix with apple cider vinegar and honey to taste. Just inhaling the odor of the horseradish as you grate will be enough to open your sinuses and relieve your headache.

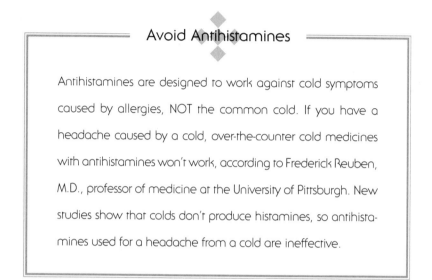

Avoid Antihistamines

Antihistamines are designed to work against cold symptoms caused by allergies, NOT the common cold. If you have a headache caused by a cold, over-the-counter cold medicines with antihistamines won't work, according to Frederick Reuben, M.D., professor of medicine at the University of Pittsburgh. New studies show that colds don't produce histamines, so antihistamines used for a headache from a cold are ineffective.

Take a Capsaicin Capsule for Headache Relief

If your head hurts because of nasal and sinus stuffiness, try taking capsaicin capsules, according to Geoffrey Watson, M.D., of Oakland, California. The capsules can ease your headache because capsaicin increases secretions of the nose and throat, unblocking congested nasal passages.

Try Goldenseal Drops

To relieve a headache associated with sinus pain, try sucking on a goldenseal drop. You can find these at most natural food stores. Goldenseal contains a powerful natural ingredient known as berberine which may stimulate the immune system, and is often combined with echinacea as a cold treatment. Some herb experts believe it stimulates the macrophages (the immune cells that engulf and destroy viruses, bacteria, and other foreign substances).

✤CAUTION: Do not take goldenseal on a daily basis, but only to fight an illness. Do not use goldenseal during pregnancy.

Relax Your Headache Away with Valerian

This so-called "nature's Valium" is very effective at relieving headaches according to herbalist experts, although researchers have not yet discovered why. Valerian is sold as capsules, tinctures, and extracts and is often combined with other herbs in various calming and insomnia formulas. The average dose is between 100 and 200 mg. of valerian extract (that contains between 0.8 and 1.0 percent valerenic acid). Because valerian root has an unpleasant smell, you may prefer the odor-free capsules instead of the liquid products.

While it is considered to be a safe herb, valerian can be so relaxing that you shouldn't take it before driving or doing tasks that require full attention—nor should you take it for more than a few weeks. A small number of people find valerian stimulating instead of relaxing.

✤CAUTION: Valerian should not be used by anyone under age 12.

For Headache Pain, Take Feverfew Capsules

This relative of the chrysanthemum family is used to reduce headache pain by preventing blood vessels from dilating. It's a favorite remedy of Annette Stoesser, M.D., of Roswell, New Mexico. While its traditional use was to reduce fevers (as you can tell by its name), it also has a long history of treating headaches.

Researchers have found that feverfew can reduce the number and severity of migraines and appears to interfere with the production of a number of chemicals that may be related to headaches, including histamines and the brain neurotransmitter serotonin. Actually how feverfew works, however, is still not fully understood.

You can buy feverfew dried, in concentrated drops, tinctures, extracts, or in capsules. The newest products have standardized doses (usually between 0.1 to 0.2 percent parthenolide, the active compound in feverfew). Herbalists recommend the average daily dose of a 0.2 percent parthenolide product to be 125 mg. of feverfew.

Side effects are rare, although if you eat the fresh leaves your mouth and tongue could become numb.

Drink Healing Teas

Some herbalists swear by the headache-relieving properties of ginger-chive tea. Here's the simple recipe:

GINGER-CHIVE TEA

1½ tablespoons minced chives
½ teaspoon shredded gingerroot

Steep chives and ginger for 30 minutes in a cup of boiling water. Strain and drink.

To relieve the pain of a virus-induced headache, try sipping chamomile tea made from a teabag, or try this recipe from dried chamomile flowers:

FRESH CHAMOMILE TEA

1 teaspoon dried chamomile flowers
1 cup hot water

Steep for 3–5 minutes; strain and drink.

Sip Chicken Soup, the Tried and True Healer

Chicken soup can cure not only generalized cold symptoms, but the headache resulting from a cold as well. It's also been proven to work better in concert with vegetables, according to Stephen Rennard, M.D., chief of pulmonary and critical care medicine at the University of Nebraska Medical Center in Omaha. Dr. Rennard tested plain chicken broth in a test tube and found it somewhat reduced the inflammation- producing activity of white blood cells, suggesting it might ease cold symptoms. When he added vegetables (onions, sweet potatoes, carrots, turnips, and parsnips) he found that the anti-inflammatory effect grew stronger.

CHICKEN SOUP

4–5 pounds of chicken

3 carrots (scrubbed or peeled), cut in thirds

2 celery stalks with leaves, cut in thirds

1 large onion, cut in half

1 green pepper, cut in half and cleaned out

2 sprigs of dill or ½ teaspoon dill seeds (optional)

4 sprigs of parsley

4 cloves of garlic, crushed

1–2 teaspoons salt

10 cups water

Combine chicken, vegetables, water, and salt in a big pot. Wrap dill or seeds, parsley, and garlic in cheesecloth, and add to pot.

Bring to boil, clean off scum from the top of the soup, cover, and simmer for 2-3 hours. If after 3 hours the soup doesn't have the flavor you want, add a few chicken bouillon cubes to taste.

Remove and reserve chicken and vegetables; refrigerate soup overnight. The next day, remove the top layer of fat from the soup before reheating, skimming the surface with a spoon. Add vegetables and chicken, and heat through.

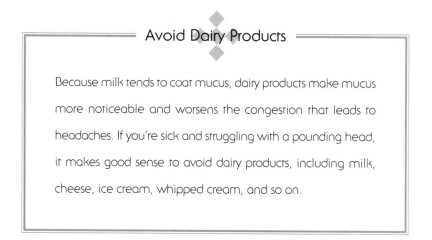

Avoid Dairy Products

Because milk tends to coat mucus, dairy products make mucus more noticeable and worsens the congestion that leads to headaches. If you're sick and struggling with a pounding head, it makes good sense to avoid dairy products, including milk, cheese, ice cream, whipped cream, and so on.

Stop Your Headache with Acupressure

Acupressure is based on the same principle as acupuncture: Key points of the body are stimulated to enhance the flow of energy to all organs and body systems. Experts trained in the art of acupressure believe that if you apply pressure to certain points, you can relieve a headache.

You may be able to rub your headache away by pressing on these acupressure points gently to the count of 5 and then releasing:

- Squeeze the web of skin between your thumb and forefinger gently.

- Squeeze the tiny ridge between your neck and the back of your head (parallel with your ear lobes).

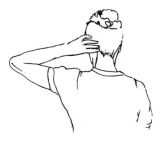

- Press down against the top peak of your foot.

- Pinch gently 1 inch out from each nostril on your cheeks and between your eyebrows.

- Press against the roof of your mouth with your thumb.

- Squeeze gently the area between your big and second toe.

- Press on the outside of your shin just below the knee.

How to Tell If Infected Sinuses Are Causing Your Headache

The following signs may indicate a sinus infection:

- Fever

- Pain lasting for more than two days

- Green or yellow nasal or postnasal discharge

If your headache is accompanied by any of these symptoms,

consult with your doctor.

Bathe in Herbs for Your Body Aches

When your whole body is aching, you can help relax joints and muscle aches in a hot bath with dry mustard or dry ginger powder, according to Donald J. Carrow, M.D., of Clearwater, Florida. Fill the tub with hot water, add ¼ cup of either dry ginger or mustard, and swirl in water to dissolve. Soak for 10 to 20 minutes.

Pack in the Hot Salt

A hot salt pack works on the same principle as a hot water bottle, bringing fresh blood to the area to ease aches. Heat a pound of salt in a heavy pan on the stove. Funnel it into a clean, heavy cotton sock. (Don't overfill; the sock should be pliable.) Pin the end securely and apply the warm sock to the painful area.

Heat It Up for Healing Relaxation

Most of the time, using heat on aches and pains when you're sick will make you feel better and relaxed. The heat dilates the blood vessels, and can promote healing. Warm baths, whirlpools, and heating pads are all good ways to ease the aches that can accompany colds.

In the Next Chapter

One of the most common symptoms of a cold is sinus congestion. For lots of effective, easy-to-use home remedies, read on!

20 Sinus
Congestion Busters

HEN YOUR NOSE becomes congested, the nasal lining swells, closing the sinuses. When the sinuses can't drain, they can become infected and turn a common cold into a sinus or middle ear infection. To avoid such complications and make yourself feel better, it's a good idea to try to relieve the congestion as soon as possible with these doctor-recommended natural remedies.

Try Hot Chicken Soup

This long-favorite folk remedy really does work, according to researchers at Mount Sinai Medical Center in Miami Beach, Florida. Hot chicken soup can unclog your nasal passages, increasing the flow of nasal mucus either because of its aroma, taste, temperature, and nutrients.

Why has everyone from the time of the celebrated 12th century physician Moses Maimonides prescribed chicken soup for stuffy noses and colds? First, it's important to drink fluids lost from breathing through your mouth. Hot liquids are better because virologists have shown that heat can kill viruses (at least in a test tube). When made traditionally, with carrots, celery, onions, parsley, garlic, and spices, chicken soup provides a good dose of vitamin A, and a raft of B vitamins—especially important when your appetite is off.

Moreover, chicken (like most proteins) contains a natural amino acid called cystine, which is released as the soup cooks. Cystine is remarkably similar to a drug called acetylcysteine, which is prescribed for respiratory infections, according to Irwin Ziment, M.D., a pulmonary specialist at UCLA. According to Dr. Ziment, acetylcysteine thins out the mucus, making it less sticky. In fact, the drug acetylcysteine was originally produced from chicken feathers and skin.

How you make chicken soup can make all the difference, Ziment insists. The hotter and spicier, the better—so include plenty of pepper, curry powder, and garlic.

SPICY CHICKEN SOUP

1 whole garlic bulb (about 15 cloves)

1 4-pound chicken

2 onions, halved

4 celery stalks with leaves, diced

4 carrots, peeled and diced

3 quarts water

1 teaspoon hot curry powder

1 teaspoon black pepper

3 teaspoons fresh basil, chopped, or 1 teaspoon dried basil

6 sprigs cilantro, minced

5 sprigs parsley, minced

salt to taste

Peel garlic and place whole into large pot with chicken and half the vegetables. Add water and spices, bring to boil, reduce heat and simmer uncovered for 2 hours.

Skim fat off the top and strain the soup. Remove the cooked chicken and refrigerate for later use.

Add remaining vegetables to the broth; simmer 10 minutes. Serve.

═══ Eliminate Dairy Foods ═══

If you want to ease a stuffy nose, avoid milk and dairy foods, according to Phyllis Stoffman, B.S.N., M.H.Sc. Research suggests that dairy products worsen nasal congestion. At least one study published in the International Archives of Allergy and Applied Immunology links milk products to an increase of histamine, a body chemical involved in causing runny noses and nasal congestion.

Spice Up Your Food

One good way to unclog stuffed nasal passages is by eating some spicy food, according to Dr. Ziment. Spicy foods trigger a release of watery fluids in your mouth, throat, and nasal passages that helps to thin mucus.

Try some of these spicy cures:

HORSERADISH DECONGESTANT CURE

½ teaspoon prepared horseradish
a few drops of lemon juice

Mix the horseradish and lemon juice together. Each morning and evening, eat a bit of this natural decongestant mixture until your nose starts to feel a bit better.

ONION DECONGESTANT CURE

1 medium sliced raw onion
1 cup water

Cover the onion with water. Let stand for 1 minute. Remove the onion and then drink the water. Repeat twice a day until congestion eases.

GARLIC DECONGESTANT CURE

If your nose is driving you crazy, throw lots of garlic into your soups, your broths, sauces—anything you can think of. In this case, it's best to use natural raw garlic in its orginal form, not garlic tablets. You're going for the spicy smell here. Garlic contains ingredients that help loosen congestion, and is probably the best recognized expectorant there is, according to Dr. Ziment.

CAJUN SPICE DECONGESTANT

While no one has done a study to see if people in New Orleans get fewer stuffy noses, health experts believe that eating lots of spicy foods that include Cajun spices can help you begin to breathe more easily through your nose. Cayenne peppers, which contain the natural decongestant capsaicin, are especially good at unblocking stuffy sinuses.

When you're cooking your sauces or chicken soup, throw in as much prepared cajun spice or cayenne pepper as you can stand. Breathe deeply as you stir the soup and as you spoon up the broth.

Take a Hot Shower

Taking a hot, steamy shower is a good way to ease your congestion. If you don't feel like taking a shower, you can try steam inhalation, according to Kenneth Peters, M.D., an internist specializing in self-care and chronic pain in Mountain View, California.

To do this, boil some water in a pot, drape a towel over your head as you bend over the pot, and inhale the steam. Repeat as often as necessary until you begin to feel better.

Sip Hot, Steaming Tea

Any kind of hot, steaming tea will help ease congestion, according to medical experts. Research suggests that the heat from the tea can help to promote mucus flow, which can loosen congestion and unclog stuffy noses.

The way to benefit the most from hot beverages is to first sniff the steam, and then drink the tea. Here are two good choices:

MINT TEA

The oil in mint is menthol, an FDA-approved decongestant used in such cold formulas as Vicks VapoRub. When used as a tea, the odor of the hot mint can help ease a stuffy nose, experts say.

1 handful or bunch of fresh mint leaves, or 2 teaspoons of dried leaves
1 cup boiling water

Steep leaves for 10 minutes in boiling water.
Drink up to 3 cups a day.

MULLEIN TEA

2 teaspoons of dried leaves
1 cup hot water

Mix together and steep for 5 minutes.

Sip Elderberry Tea

The berries and flowers of the elderberry bush can be very helpful in drying up the sniffles of a common cold, according to experts. You can buy elderberry as a tincture, an extract capsule, lozenge, syrup, liquid extract, or throat spray.

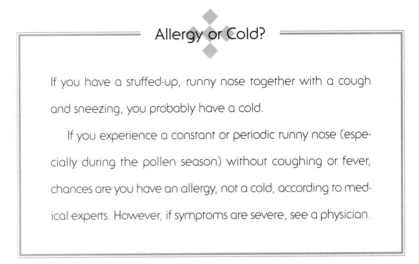

Allergy or Cold?

If you have a stuffed-up, runny nose together with a cough and sneezing, you probably have a cold.

If you experience a constant or periodic runny nose (especially during the pollen season) without coughing or fever, chances are you have an allergy, not a cold, according to medical experts. However, if symptoms are severe, see a physician.

Drink Plenty of Fluids

To make up for all that water lost during sneezing and nasal discharge, you must drink at least 2 quarts of liquid a day, according to medical experts. Fluids help thin out sticky mucus, and will loosen thick secretions. This, in turn, will help make your stuffy nose feel clearer.

Humidify Your Home

When you first turn the heat on in the fall, the atmosphere in your house probably gets extremely dry. This will only make a stuffy nose feel worse.

To keep your sinuses moist and feeling better while you are battling a cold, turn on a humidifier, according to Phyllis Stoffman. If you don't have a humidifier, you can try boiling a big pot of water on the stove, or setting pans of water under heating registers. Make sure the air in your bedroom is properly humidified.

Inhale Potent, Soothing Oils

When you're having trouble breathing due to an inflamed, congested nasal passage, aromatherapy experts suggest inhaling the following mixture on a tissue:

2 drops rosemary oil
1 drop geranium
1 drop eucalyptus

Sniffing potent or soothing oils can help shrink swollen membranes and thin mucus, easing your breathing.

Or Sniff Eucalyptus Oil by Itself

Eucalyptus oil drops are available over-the-counter at many drug stores, according to Richard Kunin, M.D., of San Francisco, California. This iodized form of eucalyptus oil is very effective in relieving nasal congestion and irritation, and preventing the development of a secondary sinus infection after the cold is over.

Sniff Saline Drops

Saline can help clear mucus from the nose. To insert, lie down on a bed with your head back; put 2 to 3 drops of saline in each nostril. Suction out using a suction bulb.

You can buy saline drops at your local pharmacy, or, even better, make your own:

SALINE SOLUTION

½ teaspoon salt
8 ounces warm water

Mix together, place 2–3 drops in each nostril, then suction out using a suction bulb.

Oil Your Nose

This remedy won't help unstop your nose, but it will help you feel better while you wait for your sinuses to clear themselves out. If your nose is sore from all that blowing, dab a layer of petroleum jelly around and a little inside the nostrils with a cotton swab, Dr. Peters advises. This is especially effective if applied right before going to bed, so the petroleum jelly will remain undisturbed on the skin for several hours.

You may also find that tissues containing lotion can help prevent reddened, irritated noses.

Take Goldenseal As an Anti-Inflammatory

Health experts believe the root of this herb can help ease chronic inflammation of the mucous membranes lining the nose and sinuses. When your body's mucous membranes become inflamed, they lose their ability to secrete mucus, which normally would trap bacteria and viruses. This means that germs can then enter the circulatory system. Scientists believe that two alkaloids in goldenseal (berberine and hydrastine) may contribute to the herb's ability to ease this inflammation.

Since goldenseal is one of the most popular herbs in the United States, overharvesting of the wild roots have led to recent shortages and boosted prices. Within 5 to 10 years, increased cultivation is expected to eliminate these shortages.

To ease a stuffy, inflamed nasal passage, take 0.5 to 1 g. of the powdered root daily. Alternatively, every 2 to 3 hours you could take 20 to 30 drops of the liquid extract or one capsule.

❖❖CAUTION: Take goldenseal only until the inflammation subsides, since the strong alkaloids could harm your liver if used for a long period of time. Do not take goldenseal at all during pregnancy, since the herb can induce contractions.

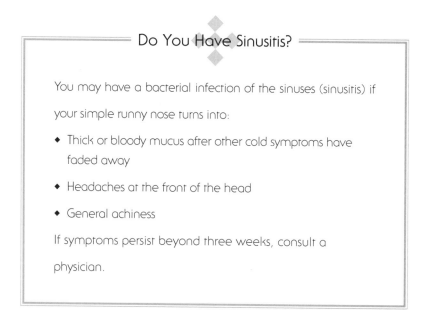

Do You Have Sinusitis?

You may have a bacterial infection of the sinuses (sinusitis) if your simple runny nose turns into:

- Thick or bloody mucus after other cold symptoms have faded away

- Headaches at the front of the head

- General achiness

If symptoms persist beyond three weeks, consult a physician.

Eat Citrus Peel, a Congestion-Buster

To ease clogged nasal passages, medical advisers suggest eating 1 teaspoon grated lemon or orange peel (plain or sweetened with honey) each morning and evening.

If eating plain peels doesn't appeal to you, try soaking small strips of orange peel in cider vinegar, drain, and cook with honey for 5–10 minutes. Eat 1 or 2 at bedtime.

Try Amylase Capsules and Bioflavonoid

To ease a stuffy nose and sinus congestion, Alan Cohen, M.D., medical director of Harmony Health Care in Milford, Connecticut, advises patients to take 2 capsules each of the digestive enzyme amylase with a bioflavonoid (lesperidin) 3 to 4 times a day on an empty stomach.

Sip Potassium Iodide, A Powerful Healer

This compound, when diluted in water or juice (about 10 drops per glass) is gentle but retains its antiseptic properties, according to Dr. Kunin. Potassium iodide is not the same as the rusty-brown common iodine, the caustic liquid used as an antiseptic. Instead, potassium iodide (available with prescription) looks like water and causes no irritation except when applied to raw or damaged tissues. It may burn, but it causes no harm, Dr. Kunin says.

Potassium iodide stimulates the immune system and also works as an antibiotic, killing most bacteria, viruses, and fungi—including the rhinovirus of the common cold. It is also a powerful antihistamine and in a matter of minutes after the first dose, Dr. Kunin says, nasal secretions usually dry up. Even those who say they have an iodine allergy can be desensitized in a day or two, according to Dr. Kunin.

Stop Sneezing with Acupressure Massage

To stop sneezing, try these doctor-recommended acupressure points:

- Press skin directly above the center of the upper lip firmly for 5 seconds just before a sneeze occurs. Release. Repeat as often as necessary.

- Press skin on the bridge of the nose firmly just before sneezing. Release after 5 seconds. Repeat as often as necessary.

Try Menthol/Camphor Rubs to Ease Congestion

The soothing effect of menthol or camphor rubs may help ease a stuffed-up nose, according to Ron Eccles, M.D., director of the Common Cold Centre in the School of Molecular and Medical Biosciences, University of Wales in Cardiff, Wales. Right before bedtime, apply Vicks VapoRub or another similar product to your chest and then cover it with a soft cloth. Breathe deeply.

Blow Your Nose to Get Rid of Germs

One of the reasons your nose runs when you have a cold is because it's the body's way of ridding itself of germs, medical experts say. Reinforce the process by blowing your nose gently and often. Don't blow too hard or blow one nostril at a time; this can force the mucus into the sinuses and ears, paving the way for a bacterial infection. It also puts too much strain on your blood vessels and lungs. The same thing can happen if your nose is swollen badly and you exert too much pressure blowing; this can force infected mucus deep into the sinuses or Eustachian tubes. For the same reason, don't routinely sniff up the mucus to clear the nose instead of blowing it out. This can be a particular problem with young children, who can develop the sniffling habit early in life.

Instead, exhale gently through both nostrils, holding a handkerchief or tissue in front of your nose but wiping as little as possible to avoid skin irritation.

Exercise to Clear Your Nose!

If you're not too sick, try some light exercise. It will act as a natural decongestant by increasing adrenaline which leads to more air flow through the nose, according to Kathleen Yaremchuk, M.D., clinical professor of otolaryngology at the University of Michigan Medical School. However, don't put yourself through a normal workout. You can't expect your body to exercise strenuously while fighting off a cold.

In the Next Chapter

In the next chapter, you'll learn a host of doctor-recommended ways to stop the nausea and vomiting that sometimes accompany other cold symptoms.

CHAPTER EIGHT

20 Quick Ways to Treat
Nausea and Vomiting

N AUSEA DOESN'T JUST involve your stomach — it's a complex reaction involving various areas of the brain as well. Nausea and vomiting occur when the vomiting center in the brain stem is activated, sending signals to the abdomen. These messages signal the diaphragm to press down on the stomach, and to contract the abdominal wall muscles; the sphincter between the stomach and the esophagus relaxes and the stomach contents are propelled upward toward the mouth.

The following 20 tips have been suggested by health experts as a way to ease your nausea naturally.

Control Your Nausea Using Acupressure and Massage

Acupressure is quick and easy to learn, according to George Milowe, M.D., a Saratoga Springs, New York psychiatrist who also practices acupuncture and Chinese herbal medicine. For conditions like nausea, it makes sense to try a little acupressure yourself in the comfort of your home.

There are six pressure points that can ease nausea, according to Leon Chaitow, N.D., D.O. You don't need to use them all; just find the one that works for you. The most effective points for nausea are:

- indentation between the earlobe and the jawbone

- 4 finger-widths above the center of the inner wrist crease, between the tendons

- middle of the inner side of the forearm, 2½ finger-widths above the wrist crease

- 4 finger-widths below the kneecap and one finger-width outside the shinbone, where the muscle flexes as the foot moves up and down

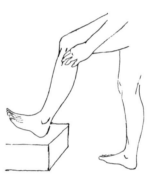

- top of the foot in the valley between the big toe and second toe

- outside of the base of the second toe

Once you think you've found the right place, probe the area with a fingertip in the general location. You'll know you've hit the right place if you feel a bit of tenderness, tingling, soreness, or minor discomfort. Press each point firmly for one minute, then stop for a few seconds before pressing again. Work each point for 5 to 20 minutes. Breathe deeply when pressing. It's best to use this method before you actually start vomiting.

If you're feeling nauseated, try firmly massaging:

- your thumbs and first and second fingers in a firm, gentle circular motion

- the webs between your thumbs and index fingers in a firm circular motion

- 1 inch to the left of the center of your chest for 10 seconds; release and then repeat 3 times

- the area between the ball of each foot and the beginning of the arch, gently in a circular motion

- the area between the second and third toes on each foot with firm, gentle, circular motion

Drink Mint Tea

One of the oldest herbal remedies for an upset stomach is a cup of mint or catnip tea made with fresh-picked herbs. Mint or catnip (or a combination of both) is soothing to the stomach and relaxing. To prepare, pick a handful of fresh herbs, place in a pot and pour hot water over to steep for 5 minutes. Sip slowly. Some people notice a numbing sensation in the throat, which is a reaction to the menthol in the plants.

You may also want to try commercially-prepared mint, chamomile, or eucalyptus tea bags.

Suck on Peppermint Candy

Hard peppermint candies or a drop of tincture of peppermint can help ease some nausea. Peppermint is an antispasmodic (muscle relaxant) whose main ingredient is menthol, relaxing the circular muscle at the base of the esophagus. It can also calm agitated muscles in the stomach.

❖❖❖CAUTION: Peppermint oil can be toxic.

Ease Nausea and Vomiting with Ginger

Ginger has been used to treat nausea for thousands of years, according to oncologist Barry Rosenbloom, M.D., at Cedars-Sinai Medical Center in Los Angeles. Anyone who has ever sipped ginger ale after vomiting has discovered the soothing effects of ginger. In fact, at least one study found that ginger relieves the nausea of motion sickness better than standard drug treatments such as Dramamine. Technically, ginger is a rhizome, or "underground stem," not a root; it appears to act not just on the stomach, but on the brain as well. It contains an essential oil and other compounds that may carry antioxidant properties. In one study, doctors found that ginger effectively prevented nausea after gynecological surgery.

You can grow ginger yourself so you'll always have some handy (see box). Or you can buy ginger in a grocery or health food store. If you buy fresh ginger, remember to refrigerate the whole root. It can also be purchased dried, in tablets, capsules, tinctures, extracts, syrups, and teas. Ginger is very safe, and can even be taken in fairly large doses without causing any side effects. Indeed, many pregnant women use ginger to help control nausea and morning sickness.

There are several good ways to ease nausea and vomiting through the use of ginger:

- Take ginger capsules: 940 mg., or about 2 standard capsules.

- Drink 3 cups of ginger tea per day. To make ginger tea, use 1 teaspoon dried ginger per cup of boiling water; steep for 10 minutes.

- Slowly sip ginger ale. Let it stand in a glass for several hours before drinking, so it becomes flat and lukewarm. Sip in tiny swallows; if you can keep a sip down, sip again. Don't drink more than an ounce or so at a time.

- Nibble on a small piece of crystallized ginger.

- If your symptoms are very mild, try slowly eating a few ginger snaps.

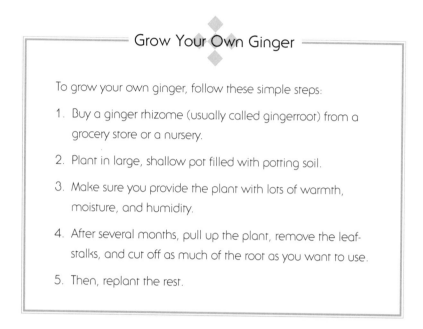

Grow Your Own Ginger

To grow your own ginger, follow these simple steps:

1. Buy a ginger rhizome (usually called gingerroot) from a grocery store or a nursery.

2. Plant in large, shallow pot filled with potting soil.

3. Make sure you provide the plant with lots of warmth, moisture, and humidity.

4. After several months, pull up the plant, remove the leaf-stalks, and cut off as much of the root as you want to use.

5. Then, replant the rest.

You'll know you've had enough when you start burping and taste ginger, according to herbal medicine researcher Daniel Mowrey, Ph.D., a psychopharmacologist in Lehi, Utah. If you don't taste any ginger in your mouth five minutes after taking a capsule, you know you haven't taken enough.

It's probably best to take ginger capsules rather than fresh ginger because the fresh variety may be too strong for most people. Some people find that ginger causes heartburn. If this happens to you, discontinue use.

If you are pregnant, check with your physician before using ginger capsules.

Sip Chamomile Tea to Calm Your Stomach

Chamomile has a long history as a digestive aid, and scientific studies have supported this claim. The flower heads of the German chamomile (*Matricaria recutita*) and Roman chamomile (*Chamaemelum*

117

nobile) have been used as a way to soothe an upset stomach for centuries.

Several chemicals in chamomile oil seem to relax the muscles of the stomach and intestinal wall. In addition, its flavonoids reduce inflammation and stimulate the immune-boosting activities of white blood cells. German chamomile seems to be more effective than Roman chamomile at reducing inflammation.

If you're feeling nauseated or are vomiting, drink a cup of chamomile tea to calm the stomach. You can buy chamomile tea at any supermarket or health food store. To make your own, combine 2 or 3 heaping teaspoons of dried chamomile blossoms to a cup of boiling water; steep for 10–20 minutes.

Avoid chamomile—a member of the daisy family—if you are allergic to ragweed, aster, or chrysanthemums, because it may trigger an allergic reaction. While this reaction is rare, it does occasionally occur. For the vast majority of people, chamomile products are considered to be quite nontoxic and gentle enough for children and pregnant or breastfeeding women.

Brew Up Some Clove Tea

Clove tea is another effective remedy for nausea. Here's how you make it:

10 whole cloves
1 cup hot water

Try steeping the whole cloves in boiling water for 5 minutes. If you find the taste unpleasant, add a piece of cinnamon stick to the cloves and steep together. Sip slowly.

Chew a Natural Cure

Try one of these chewable remedies to offset nausea and vomiting:

- 1 or 2 whole cloves
- ½ teaspoon dry grated grapefruit peel
- fresh mint leaves
- fresh sage leaves
- fresh catnip leaves (plants are sold at most nurseries and herbal shops)

Try Valerian, Nature's Valium

Valerian, sometimes called "nature's Valium," is also a good way to calm a nervous stomach, according to herb experts. Prepared from the rhizome and roots of Valeriana officinalis, it now grows throughout the northeastern United States. A very effective sleep-promoter, it may interact with certain brain receptors in ways that have a calming effect on the body.

Valerian is found as a capsule, tincture, or extract and is often combined with other calming herbs in various herbal preparations. Because of the unpleasant smell of the liquid, most people prefer to use this herb in its capsule form. An average dose is between 100 mg. and 200 mg. containing 0.8 to 1.0 percent valerenic acid.

Try a Vitamin B6 Tablet

Some people find that 25 mg. of vitamin B6 every 8 hours works to help stop nausea and vomiting. Most doctors recommend that you take no more than 50 mg. a day of vitamin B6 without medical supervision.

❖❖❖CAUTION: Very high doses of vitamin B6 can be harmful, and long-term use of high doses has been associated with nerve damage.

Mom Was Right: Cola Syrup Works!

If you're mildly nauseated, you might try the old standby: cola syrup, according to pharmacist Robert Warren at Valley Children's Hospital in Fresno, California. Scientists believe that the noncarbonated syrup has concentrated carbohydrates that may account for its anti-nausea properties. Actually, any soft drink syrup — or just plain sugar syrup — should also work.

To try it out, take 1 to 2 tablespoons for adults (room temperature) and 1 to 2 teaspoons for children.

Don't Forget to Drink Clear Fluids

Doctors agree that it's essential to avoid becoming dehydrated from vomiting by drinking plenty of fluids. To avoid insulting an upset stomach further, stick to clear liquids such as tea and juice, according to nausea researcher Kenneth Koch, M.D., a gastroenterologist at Hershey Medical Center in Hershey, Pennsylvania.

Be sure to drink no more than 1 or 2 ounces at a time at room temperature. If you drink too fast, your stomach will distend and your nausea will return.

If you're going to drink clear carbonated beverages such as ginger ale, let the glass sit out until it becomes flat and lukewarm. Remember to sip in tiny swallows, not enormous gulps. Don't drink more than an ounce or so at a time. How often you can sip depends on how your stomach reacts; if you can keep a sip down, you can sip again.

Try to get to the point where you're drinking at least 6 to 8 ounces an hour. A good way to tell if you're getting enough fluids is by the frequency and color of your urine. If you urinate frequently and the color is light yellow, your water balance is normal.

If you can't even stomach water, try sucking on ice cubes or ice chips. They can make you feel better, although it's not likely that just doing this will provide you with enough fluids.

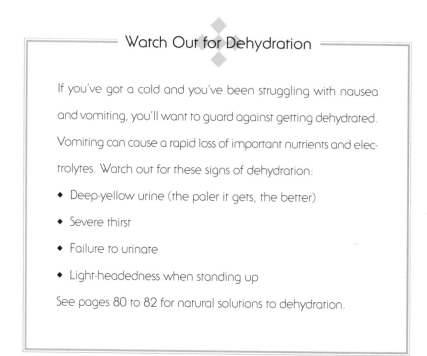

Watch Out for Dehydration

If you've got a cold and you've been struggling with nausea and vomiting, you'll want to guard against getting dehydrated. Vomiting can cause a rapid loss of important nutrients and electrolytes. Watch out for these signs of dehydration:

- Deep-yellow urine (the paler it gets, the better)
- Severe thirst
- Failure to urinate
- Light-headedness when standing up

See pages 80 to 82 for natural solutions to dehydration.

Reach for an Electrolyte Drink

If you're vomiting, you're not just losing fluids—you're losing valuable minerals as well. Taking electrolyte drinks will help replace these nutrients (the sodium, potassium, chloride, and bicarbonate elements that your body needs to function). Examples of electrolyte drinks include Pedialyte (which may taste terrible) and Gatorade. New on the market are Pedialyte flavored popsicles. They may not taste exactly like the real thing, but they are often a good choice for a young child who balks at the flavor of traditional Pedialyte. You can buy them at your pharmacy and keep them frozen until needed.

Clear soups, or apple or cranberry juice are good choices to sip every half hour, according to Samuel Klein, M.D., assistant professor of gastroenterology and human nutrition at the University of Texas

Medical School at Galveston. While water is better than no fluid at all, it's better to add some salt and sugar to each glass.

Drink Your Bitters

To ease an upset stomach and stop vomiting, try drinking 1 table-spoon of bitters (alone or poured over ice), according to Curt Kurtz, M.D., of Bozeman, Montana. You can find bitters in the "drink mix" section of most grocery stores. According to Dr. Kurtz, bitters is not harmful, even to children.

Eat Light Carbohydrates for Strength and Energy

Most likely you won't feel like eating much if your stomach is upset, and in fact, you should give your stomach a chance to rest. But if you do need to eat a little something, try small amounts of light carbo-hydrates—saltines or toast, for example.

Carbohydrates are usually well tolerated and more easily digested by an upset stomach, and may give you strength and energy when you haven't eaten for a long period of time. As you begin to feel better, move on to some light protein—physicians usually recommend chicken breast or light fish.

Doctors Recommend the Brat Diet

Eight hours after you've stopped vomiting, you should be able to tol-erate the BRAT diet (bananas, rice, applesauce, and toast). Bananas contain electrolytes, and they are soft and easy to digest. Rice is filled with carbohydrates and is a bit constipating (a boon if you've been having loose stools). Applesauce is easy to digest and provides some sugar for energy, and the toast will provide bulk for the stomach.

Other foods that are well tolerated by an upset stomach on the mend are scrambled eggs, pasta, and broth. If you're a dedicated milk drinker, a week after you've vomited you can start with skim milk and move gradually on to 1 or 2 percent, and then whole milk. It takes this long because the enzyme that metabolizes milk is located on the superficial surface of the intestine. Vomiting destroys this enzyme, which will interfere with your ability to digest milk.

Eat That Ultimate Comfort Food: Jello

If you want to try eating something that won't upset your stomach, reach for mild-flavored Jello. It's the traditional choice hospitals use to introduce food to someone who's been vomiting.

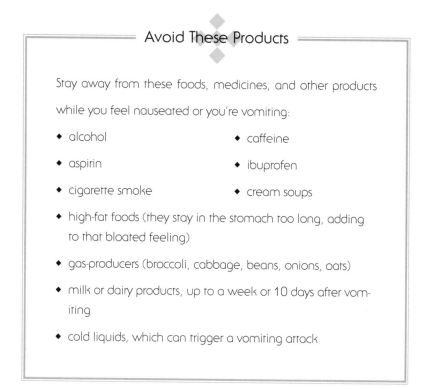

Avoid These Products

Stay away from these foods, medicines, and other products while you feel nauseated or you're vomiting:

- alcohol
- caffeine
- aspirin
- ibuprofen
- cigarette smoke
- cream soups
- high-fat foods (they stay in the stomach too long, adding to that bloated feeling)
- gas-producers (broccoli, cabbage, beans, onions, oats)
- milk or dairy products, up to a week or 10 days after vomiting
- cold liquids, which can trigger a vomiting attack

Put on a Hot Pack

Place one of these hot packs over your bare stomach and keep warm with a heating pad:

- washcloth saturated with cinnamon tea
- washcloth saturated with vinegar
- poultice of crushed mint leaves wrapped in moistened cloth

...Or Try a Cold Pack

If heat doesn't work, you can try the opposite. Applying an ice pack against the back of your neck, or a cool cloth against your forehead, can sometimes ease a churning stomach.

When All Else Fails—You Can Always Vomit

One of the most effective ways to cure nausea is to allow yourself to vomit. If it doesn't cure the nausea, it will probably bring you some temporary relief from that ill-at-ease feeling, according to Steven Lamm, M.D., assistant clinical professor of medicine at New York University School of Medicine in New York City.

However, experts don't recommend that you make yourself throw up; just allow it to happen naturally. If you're feeling nauseated enough, it probably will.

In the Next Chapter

Coughing can be an annoying symptom of the common cold, especially if your stuffy nose is causing your sinuses to drip down the back of your throat. To learn about a variety of natural ways to ease your cough, read on!

36 Ways to
Stop a Cough

 DDS ARE if you have a cold, you're also coughing due to inflammation of the upper respiratory tract (the throat, voice box, and windpipe). A cough is your body's response to this irritation in the throat, larynx, bronchial tubes, or lungs.

There are two specific types of coughs — productive and nonproductive. The most common type of cough associated with the common cold is a nonproductive cough. This type of cough is dry and scratchy, and doesn't produce any sputum.

A productive cough brings up sputum from the respiratory tract. When you do this, you will recover quicker. Therefore, anything you can do to loosen the mucus in the lungs and cough it up will make you feel better. This is why you don't want to suppress productive coughs with cough medicine.

The good news is that eventually, even if you don't treat the cough, it will probably fade away within two weeks. However, there are good reasons to try to break the coughing reflex. Night coughs can interfere with sleep, which you need to recover from a cold. More seriously, prolonged coughing spells can be painful and, if severe enough, can even cause you to break a rib. Read on for effective natural remedies that will ease a nagging cough.

Suck on Zinc

Recent studies suggest that if you use zinc lozenges, you may get over your cough three days sooner than you would have otherwise. The most recent study of zinc looked at lemon-flavored zinc gluconate lozenges sold under the name "Cold-eeze." While plain zinc has a very bad taste, flavored lozenges are more palatable. Many people swear by the benefits of sucking on zinc in the form of one of these lemon-flavored lozenges.

Or Try Other Types of Lozenges

If you have a dry cough, you may find relief by sucking on a variety of lozenges or hard candies. Cough drops may help (although they contain no medicine) by coating the mouth with saliva, which can ease the tickle in the throat associated with setting off a cough.

In addition, cough drops and lozenges may also help bring increased blood flow to the bronchial linings, easing a cough, according to Stephen Rayle, M.D., staff physician at St. Mary's Hospital in Tucson, Arizona. Lozenges containing licorice, aromatic oils (peppermint or spearmint), or horehound are particularly good.

Lozenges work so well in easing coughs that the Omaha Symphony in Nebraska hands out free cough drops in the lobby during winter concerts.

Drink Up!

Drinking plenty of water, fruit juice, or carbonated beverages (ginger ale is best) can help loosen and thin out mucus, according to Edward Garrity, Jr., M.D., director of the Pulmonary Function Lab at the Loyola University Medical Center.

Other good juice choices include fresh carrot or cherry juice made half-and-half with honey, or hot grapefruit juice sweetened with honey. Or try ⅔ cup lemon juice simmered with ½ pound brown sugar and a tablespoon of almond oil.

Plan to drink at least 6 glasses of fluid a day. Avoid caffeine or alcoholic beverages; they are diuretics and will lead to the loss of fluids.

Brew a Warm Drink

Warm, soothing drinks can often soothe an irritated, inflamed throat and ease the cough reflex, according to Anthony Yonkers, M.D., professor and chair of the Department of Otolaryngology–Head and Neck Surgery at the University of Nebraska Medical Center in Omaha. The steam loosens thick mucus which helps control coughing.

Some swear by the soothing properties of peppermint tea. However, when made from fresh peppermint, you may experience a choking sensation from the menthol, according to Varro Tyler, Ph.D., professor of pharmacognosy at the School of Pharmacy and Pharmacal Sciences at Purdue University. It won't hurt you, although some say peppermint tea should not be given to infants and young children for this reason.

Take a Hot Bath

If you have a dry cough, try taking several hot showers or baths a day to cleanse waste products from your body. As you shower or bathe, inhale the steam to help loosen congestion in your lungs so you can cough out the mucus, according to Dr. Garrity.

If you don't feel like taking a bath, you can inhale the steam from a boiling pan of water. For an added boost, add 1 teaspoon tincture of benzoin per pint of steaming water in a bowl. Drape a towel over your head and breathe the vapors. (Benzoin can be found in drug stores.) You can also try adding mentholatum to the water for an added boost, according to James Schuler, M.D., of Smith River, California.

Vaporize

If you have a winter cold and your home is dry and overheated, a vaporizer or humidifier in the room can add moisture to the air and ease your cough, according to Dr. Garrity. This is particularly important when you sleep. A vaporizer works because humidified air helps to thin the mucus in the lungs, making your cough more productive. Adding a few drops of peppermint or spearmint oil to the vaporizer water can help liquefy phlegm.

Keep in mind that vaporizers must be kept scrupulously clean. Otherwise, they can harbor harmful bacteria and fungi that can worsen a cough. Clean the machine regularly and keep it properly maintained.

Calm Your Cough With a Camphor/Menthol Chest Rub

Another old favorite, this gentle rub (available in health stores and pharmacies) helps calm a persistent cough, especially at night, according to Dr. Schuler. Smooth the ointment on your chest, and cover with a flannel cloth. Wash the ointment off the next day.

❖❖CAUTION: Never take any chest rub internally; it's strictly a topical treatment.

Pick a Plaster

Your mother loved this remedy, and many health practitioners still believe it may help ease a cough. Place a mustard/ginger powder plaster on your chest to relieve a chest cold or deep cough. (Occasionally you may notice a skin irritation, which may burn for 5 or 10 minutes. The red irritation will subside in a few minutes.)

You also can try a poultice made of slippery elm bark. Native Americans have been using the inner portion of the slippery elm bark as a treatment for coughs for hundreds of years. (See page 130 for beverages made of slippery elm bark.)

MUSTARD/GINGER PLASTER

1 teaspoon mustard powder
1 teaspoon dry ginger powder
1–2 tablespoons olive oil

Combine ingredients, rub into chest and back. Put on an old T-shirt (this mixture stains!) and take a shower the next day.

SLIPPERY ELM POULTICE

powdered bark
water

Mix bark and water to make a paste. Apply to your chest, covering it with a cloth. Change daily.

Call the Doctor If...

- Coughing brings up yellow, brown, or green mucus

- Coughing brings up blood-tinged or bright red mucus

- You cough for more than three days for no obvious reason, or the cough doesn't get better within two weeks. A persistent cough is sometimes a symptom of serious disease.

- Coughing is accompanied by fever, skin rash, thick sputum, earache, chest pain, shortness of breath, lethargy, tooth pain, sinus pain, or confusion.

Sip Slippery Elm Bark

Native Americans have been using the inner portion of the slippery elm bark as a treatment for coughs since before the Colonists first landed, and it became a favorite cough remedy during the 18th and 19th centuries. When the great elm forests covered the east, the remedy was always handy; it was ground and mixed with milk to ease coughs. Although Dutch elm disease has decimated the forests, the bark is still available in health food stores in bulk, and in herbal cough drops and lozenges.

You can make a variety of beverages and poultices with the powder. Here are a few recipes to try:

SLIPPERY ELM BEVERAGE

1–3 teaspoons powdered bark
1 cup water

Add bark to 2 teaspoons of water to blend and avoid lumpiness.
Add remainder of water, bring to a boil, and simmer for 15 minutes.
Drink up to 3 cups a day.

SLIPPERY ELM COUGH SYRUP

1 tablespoon slippery elm powder
1 tablespoon boiling water
1/2 cup honey

Blend powder into water until dissolved; then stir into honey.
Sip for cough.

Make Your Own Cough Syrup

Natural herbal syrups are at least as effective in easing persistent coughs as any over-the-counter cough preparation, and they don't cause unwanted side effects. Here are a few favorites recommended by health experts:

RASPBERRY LEAF SYRUP

4 tablespoons dry raspberry tea

1 cup water

2 tablespoons honey

1 tablespoon lemon juice

Simmer raspberry tea in water until reduced by half. Strain. Mix the strained liquid with honey and lemon.

ANISE/THYME SYRUP

1 teaspoon anise seed

1 teaspoon dried thyme

1 teaspoon horehound (if desired)

1 teaspoon licorice root (if desired)

2 cups water

1 cup brown sugar or honey

Simmer together for 10 minutes. Strain. Stir brown sugar or honey into hot liquid. Take by teaspoon as needed for cough.

PEPPER SYRUP

½ teaspoon cayenne pepper

2 tablespoons honey

¼ cup apple cider vinegar

¼ cup water

Stir pepper and honey into vinegar and water. Take 1 teaspoon as needed.

HORSERADISH MUSTARD SYRUP

1 tablespoon horseradish
1 tablespoon crushed mustard seeds
1 cup boiling water
honey (as needed)

Steep horseradish and mustard seeds in boiling water for 20 minutes. Strain. Stir in enough honey to make a syrup. Take 1 teaspoon as needed.

Smell Your Way to Health

An offshoot of herbal medicine, aromatherapy is the science of smell, and works on the theory that smells can affect our health. Aromatherapists use many of the same aromatic oils used by herbalists. Research suggests that essential oils can be effective for a variety of ailments.

For a cough, add 3 drops of eucalyptus oil and 2 drops of thyme to 2 teaspoons of vegetable oil. Massage this mixture into your neck and chest. The old-fashioned cure for coughs and congestion—Vicks VapoRub—is basically a type of aromatherapy product that derives its decongestant vapors from eucalyptus oil.

Ease Your Cough with Licorice

Few things can soothe a cough quite like licorice, that super-sweet relative of the pea family that has been used by the Chinese, Greeks, and Europeans for centuries to treat coughs and bronchial congestion. What these ancient healers knew is that licorice root, today available at health food stores, is a natural sedative and anesthetic.

Available in a variety of products as a powder, capsule, lozenge, concentrated drop, tincture, or extract, its medicinal properties are due to glycyrrhizin (or glycyrrhizic acid, a well-known and effective cough suppressant). Unfortunately, taking high or continuous doses of glycyrrhizin may lead to problems of salt and water retention, and

high blood pressure. For this reason, people with kidney or heart problems should not take regular doses of products containing this compound. Chewable tablets and other licorice products intended for
long-term use contain just a trace of glycyrrhizin (usually 2 percent
or less); these products are known as deglycyrrhizinated licorice
(DGL), and they cause far fewer side effects.

If your cough is troubling you, try drinking a few cups of licorice
root tea a day. This tea soothes throats and eases coughing spasms,
according to Timothy Van Ert, M.D., a private practitioner and preventive medicine specialist in San Francisco and Saratoga, California.

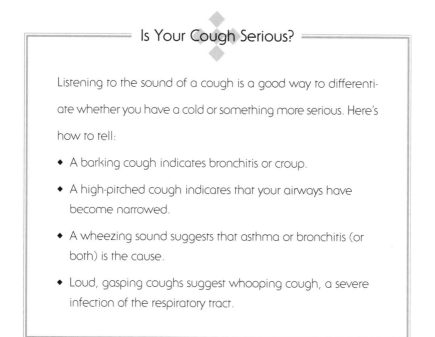

Is Your Cough Serious?

Listening to the sound of a cough is a good way to differenti-
ate whether you have a cold or something more serious. Here's
how to tell:

* A barking cough indicates bronchitis or croup.

* A high-pitched cough indicates that your airways have
  become narrowed.

* A wheezing sound suggests that asthma or bronchitis (or
  both) is the cause.

* Loud, gasping coughs suggest whooping cough, a severe
  infection of the respiratory tract.

Try Ginkgo, an Ancient Cough Remedy

One of the most well-researched of all the medicinal herbs, the long-
living Ginkgo biloba tree is known as a living fossil, having survived
almost unchanged for more than 150 million years. Among its other

uses, the Chinese have used it for thousands of years to treat coughs.

It is available as a liquid, or in an extract form as a capsule standardized to 24 percent of active ingredients. Average dose of the extract is between 40 and 60 mg. It is also sold as a powdered whole herb.

While ginkgo is considered to be safe, with few side effects and no long-term toxicity, herbalists note that those who first take the herb in doses over 300 mg. may experience headaches or stomach problems.

Suck on a Whole Clove

Sucking on a whole clove is often effective at easing a bad cough. It's tart, but worth the minor discomfort! Within minutes, you should be able to quiet that irritating tickle that sets off a cough.

Spread on Chinese Mustard

To help liquefy bronchial secretions, try eating some hot Chinese mustard, freshly prepared horseradish, and wasabi (Japanese horseradish). Andrew Weil, M.D., recommends that you eat as much as you can tolerate. Dr. Weil is associate director of the Division of Social Perspectives in Medicine at the University of Arizona College of Medicine/Arizona Health Sciences Center in Tucson.

Chew on Gingerroot

Another way to liquefy bronchial secretions is to chew on a piece of gingerroot as you would chew on a piece of gum. When you swallow the juice, you can control your cough.

Relieve Your Cough with Marsh Mallow

Real marsh mallow is a long-rooted herb that has been used for hundreds of years to stop coughing. In Germany, marsh mallow teas are commonly sold as cough suppressants.

While not widely available in the United States, some health food stores carry marsh mallow tea or crushed marsh mallow root. The flowers, roots, and leaves of the plant all contain a thick, gooey substance called mucilage that swells and becomes slippery as it absorbs water. The marsh mallow herb has nothing to do with the fluffy white marshmallows that swim in your cocoa, so don't try substituting the two. (At one time, the plant was used to make the fluffy marshmallows, but today marshmallows contain no plant material.)

To make a marsh mallow tea, boil for 10 to 15 minutes:

½–1 teaspoon crushed marsh mallow root
1 cup water

Sip slowly as needed.

Sip Some Mullein

This herbal remedy for coughing also contains mucilage, which accounts for its soothing effect on the throat. It can be taken as a tincture in doses of ½ to 1 teaspoon up to 3 times a day.

As a tea, use 1 to 2 teaspoons dried leaves per cup; allow to steep for 10 minutes. You can drink up to 3 cups per day. Because of its bitter taste, you may want to add sugar or honey for sweetness.

The U.S. Food and Drug Administration includes mullein on its list of GRAS herbs (herbs that are "generally recognized as safe"). While the seeds of the plant are toxic, there have been no reports of poisoning with leaves, flowers, or roots.

Mix Up Onions and Sugar

A popular remedy during the Depression years, onion and sugar is said to be effective in easing coughs. This may be because onions and the stimulating effect of sugar boosts the secretions of salivary glands, according to Dr. Yonkers. These secretions lubricate your mouth, minimizing your cough.

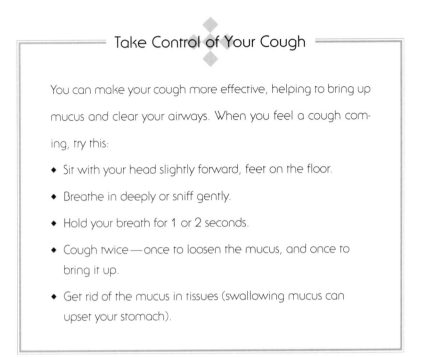

Take Control of Your Cough

You can make your cough more effective, helping to bring up mucus and clear your airways. When you feel a cough coming, try this:

♦ Sit with your head slightly forward, feet on the floor.

♦ Breathe in deeply or sniff gently.

♦ Hold your breath for 1 or 2 seconds.

♦ Cough twice—once to loosen the mucus, and once to bring it up.

♦ Get rid of the mucus in tissues (swallowing mucus can upset your stomach).

In addition, German scientists have identified several ingredients in onions that can produce anti-inflammatory effects strong enough to head off asthma attacks.

To get your onion benefits, try this: Slice two medium onions, sprinkle with sugar and cook over low heat. After 30 minutes, take 1 spoonful of the juice that seeps out every few hours.

Another recipe calls for chopping an onion into a bowl and covering it with half a cup of white sugar. Marinate overnight. The sugar absorbs liquid from the onion, creating a clear syrup. One tablespoon every 4 or 5 hours can ease a cough.

Lick Your Cough with Lemons

Whether you gargle with it, suck on it, pour it into tea, or squeeze it into a spoonful of honey, the sour yellow lemon is a popular remedy for coughs. Lemons stimulate the glands that lubricate your mouth and throat, easing the tickle that sets off a cough. Squeeze them into water, honey, tea, or whiskey, or suck on lemon candies or lozenges for maximum benefit.

Gargle Away Your Cough

Gargling with warm salt water will help bring soothing relief to your throat and respiratory tract, easing a cough. Several other gargle mixtures can also relieve a cough, and may be more palatable than the salt water.

LEMON GARGLE

4 ounces warm water

¼ cup fresh lemon juice

Combine, and gargle with mixture 3 to 4 times a day.

CORN SYRUP GARGLE

3 tablespoons dark corn syrup

8 ounces water

Mix the corn syrup with water, and gargle every hour.

Try Alcohol in Small Doses

Alcohol is used in many over-the-counter cough and cold preparations, according to Dr. Rayle, in part because in small doses it can kill bacteria and acts as a counterirritant in the esophagus. Keep in mind, however, that alcohol can increase nasal congestion. If this is a problem, skip the alcohol. Whiskey (especially combined with lemon, honey, or peppermint) is a popular cough remedy for adults.

WHISKEY REMEDY

1 teaspoon white sugar

a few drops of whiskey

Drip the whiskey on top of the sugar and swallow. The cough should stop immediately.

HOT TODDY

1 tablespoon butter

3 tablespoons whiskey

1 cup boiling water

Add butter and whiskey to water; drink as hot as possible.

MULLED WINE

3 cups wine

1-inch piece of stick cinnamon

1 tablespoon honey

3–6 cloves

3 pieces lemon peel

Heat and stir together. Drink 3 cups per day for cough.

Squirt Some Saline Solution

By squirting a saline solution up each nostril, you will rehydrate the mucous membranes of a dried-out nose to reduce coughing. You can buy a ready-to-use preparation at a drug store, or make your own: Stir 1 teaspoon of salt into 2½ cups of warm water; pour a small amount into your hand and inhale into your nose.

Take Vitamin C for Your Cough

While still controversial, many health experts swear by this vitamin, which can be effective in reducing coughs. High doses of vitamin C tablets taken for a short time shouldn't cause problems (such as diarrhea). Alternatively, you can drink orange, cranberry, or grapefruit juice, which are all high in vitamin C and will not only help your cough, but other cold symptoms as well.

Stop Your Cough with Acupressure and Massage

To stop a fit of coughing, try any of these acupressure points and massage techniques. Hold the pressure for 5 seconds, and then release.

- Squeeze the joint nearest the tip of the middle finger with the fingers of the other hand.

- Press both sides of the right thumbnail.

- Press or massage the lower joint of the right index finger.

- Press upward on the roof of the mouth.

- With the index fingers, press inward and upward against the underside of the cheekbones just above the nostrils for 30 seconds.

- Press in and pull down on the top of the breastbone at the hollow of the throat for 30 seconds.

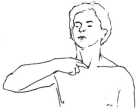

- Massage in a circular motion the hollow beneath the collarbone on both sides for 30 seconds, then firmly press the center of the breastbone.

- Press firmly the upper lip below the nose.

Visualize Your Cough Away

You can use relaxation and guided imagery to help overcome a persistent cough, according to Karen Olness, M.D., professor of pediatrics at the Case Western Reserve Medical Center in Cleveland, Ohio.

Visualization isn't difficult, but it may take practice to learn how to relax. First, find a quiet spot away from the noise and bustle of work or family. Sit in a comfortable chair, or lie down—the key is to be relaxed and comfortable. Close your eyes, breathe deeply, and count backwards from 10 to 1, very slowly. Some people imagine each number floating down past them on a cloud as they mentally count backwards. As you breathe and count, you will drift into a state of deep relaxation. Bring to your mind's eye the image of a natural scene that you find soothing: a deserted ocean beach, a deep primeval forest, an open, sunny pasture. Concentrate on soothing smells, sounds, and feelings. As you relax, your cough should ease.

Raise Your Pillows

Coughs often get worse at night when you're lying flat, allowing the lungs to fill with fluid or mucus. You can ease your breathing and stop a cough by adding a few extra pillows in bed so that your chest and head are elevated. Make sure your entire body from the waist up is raised, not just your head. Sometimes lying on your side instead of your back can also help to ease a persistent cough.

Don't Smoke!

It may seem obvious, but if you smoke, try to stop at least while you have a cold. Smoking will only aggravate your inflamed respiratory tract and worsen your cough.

If you don't smoke but you live with someone who does, try to get him or her to stop—at least while you're coughing.

In the Next Chapter

Kids and colds seem to go hand-in-hand. There are many natural ways to ease the annoying symptoms of a cold in your youngster. Read on to find out what the experts recommend.

CHAPTER TEN

The 15 Best Remedies
for Kids With Colds

OU CAN HELP PREVENT COLDS in children by following the suggestions about cold prevention for adults given earlier in this book. However, it's a fact of life that kids are going to get lots of colds. Because their immune systems are immature, they can't fight off germs as efficiently as adults, and since they are young they haven't encountered the vast variety of cold viruses that adults have, and haven't built up any immunities. Moreover, sitting in day care and elementary schools, kids are surrounded by other kids' germs—and because kids are kids, they tend to engage in risky behaviors. They put contaminated items in their mouths, they don't cover their mouths or noses when sneezing and coughing, they don't blow their noses and properly dispose of tissues.

Given the inevitable, here are a range of remedies that work well with children.

Congestion

It can be particularly difficult for a young child to cope with a stuffy nose. Infants pose particular problems, since feeding can be especially hard—it is almost impossible to suck from a bottle or breast while breathing through the mouth.

Keeping the air in your child's room humidified will soothe an inflamed nose and throat, and counteract the dryness of the air. It's particularly valuable in treating a dry, tight cough. The best way to do this, doctors agree, is with a cool-mist humidifier. An electric steam vaporizer can also get moisture into the air, but it is less efficient and less comfortable, since it also heats up the room.

To ease an infant's stuffy nose, use an infant nasal aspirator (a rubber bulb with a plastic siphon) to remove mucus and clear the nasal passages, especially just before feeding. There are a number of other things you can do to help ease your child's stuffy nose. Try these tips:

1. Use salt water nose drops instead of nasal decongestant drugs. Mix together ½ teaspoon of salt with 8 ounces of warm water, and place 2 to 3 drops in each nostril. Then suction out using a suction bulb.

2. Put the child to sleep in a right angle position to facilitate nasal drainage.

3. Raise the head of the crib (use a board under the crib legs, for example) to lessen congestion instead of propping the baby's head with a pillow.

General Cold Symptoms

Vitamin C can help ease generalized cold symptoms in children as well as adults. But if you want to give your young child vitamin C, experts don't recommend giving more than 60 mg. because it tends to cause an upset stomach and diarrhea.

Fever

Fever can have serious effects in very young children. In rare cases, a high fever can cause convulsions, coma, and even death in some situations. Remember, however, that it is quite common for children between the ages of one and five to develop a fever as high as 104 degrees F with the beginning of a mild cold just as often as with a

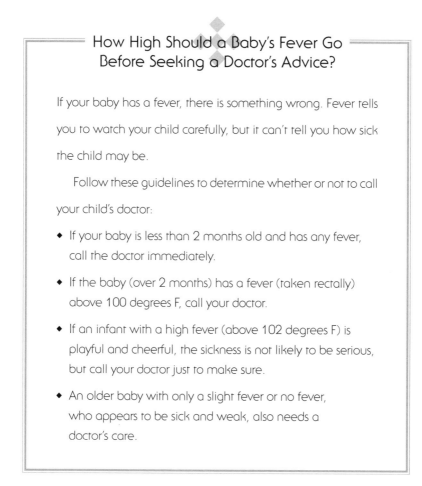

How High Should a Baby's Fever Go Before Seeking a Doctor's Advice?

If your baby has a fever, there is something wrong. Fever tells you to watch your child carefully, but it can't tell you how sick the child may be.

Follow these guidelines to determine whether or not to call your child's doctor:

• If your baby is less than 2 months old and has any fever, call the doctor immediately.

• If the baby (over 2 months) has a fever (taken rectally) above 100 degrees F, call your doctor.

• If an infant with a high fever (above 102 degrees F) is playful and cheerful, the sickness is not likely to be serious, but call your doctor just to make sure.

• An older baby with only a slight fever or no fever, who appears to be sick and weak, also needs a doctor's care.

serious infection. But fever that begins after a cold is well under way is quite a different thing—it usually means that the cold has spread, or become worse. Make sure your doctor sees your child again to rule out infections of the ear, bronchial tubes, and urinary tract. In addition to treating the underlying cause, you can try to bring down a child's fever with sponge baths, herbal teas, and by lightly covering your child.

SPONGE BATHS

Sponge the child all over with lukewarm water (NEVER alcohol, which can be absorbed by the skin or inhaled). Do not immerse a child in cold water as a way to quickly bring down a fever. Undress the child and cover him only with a light sheet. Wet your hands in lukewarm water; expose one arm and rub it gently for a couple of minutes. Put it back under the sheet. Then do the other arm, each leg, the chest and back. The rubbing brings the blood to the surface and the water cools the body by evaporation off the skin. Take the child's temperature again in half an hour; if it hasn't gone down, give cold fluids by mouth.

Febrile Seizures

Many children have a seizure at some time as a result of a high fever. Children with high fevers may be especially prone to developing febrile seizures. The child may lose consciousness or twitch for a few minutes. Make sure any dangerous objects are cleared away.

These seizures can be prevented by cooling your child's entire body as soon as the fever starts, either in a lukewarm bath or by sponging with lukewarm water.

To make sure the seizures don't return, try to reduce your child's fever using the remedies on pages 144–147.

HERBAL TEAS

Give a child peppermint, elder flower, or even yarrow tea to help the body cope with fever, according to David Hoffmann, past president of the American Herbalist Guild in Sebastopol, California. Brew the tea the same way you would for an adult, and let the child sip at will. To improve flavor, you could add a little honey. Don't give a child under age one honey because of the risk of botulism.

COVERING LIGHTLY

If your child's fever is very high, use only light covers at ordinary room temperature, or just a sheet if that's comfortable for your child. You can't reduce a fever if your child is too heavily covered.

Coughing

In order to help a child with a cough, here are some tips from nurse Phyllis Stoffman, B.S.N,. M.H.SC, and author of *The Family Guide to Preventing and Treating 100 Infectious Illnesses*:

* Loosen thick congestion by humidifying the air with a cool mist vaporizer; this will soothe an irritated respiratory tract.

* Drink lots of warm fluids to thin secretions, including clear chicken or beef broth, weak tea with honey, or apple cider. Do not give honey to an infant under age one.

* Suck on lozenges to ease the cough and provide fluids.

❖❖❖CAUTION: Do not give a child any cough medicine with codeine that has been prescribed for an adult, because it can trigger serious side effects and interfere with breathing. Instead, try one of the natural homemade remedies provided in Chapter 9. Never give a child a homemade cough syrup with alcohol.

When to Take Your Baby to the Doctor

It may look just like a common cold, but even a cold in a young baby can make new parents worry. How to tell if your baby's cold deserves a doctor visit? If your baby has any of the following symptoms, call your doctor:

- Listlessness—less alert than usual, floppier than usual, unusually sleepy or difficult to wake

- Poor feeding—not interested in nursing, refuses the bottle or breast

- Vomiting—projectile vomiting or vomiting all of the feeding (spitting up a small amount is not serious)

- Diarrhea—loose, watery, green-colored, or foul-smelling stools passed more than two or three times in a day (as opposed to formed soft stools, even if very frequent)

- Rectal temperature over 100.4 degrees F

- Convulsions

- Color changes (dark or bluish as opposed to normal skin color)

- Bulging of soft spot. If the soft spot on the baby's scalp is bulging, you can't feel the bony edges of the skull because of increased pressure in the fluid around the brain. This is a symptom of meningitis; your baby needs to see a doctor immediately.

Vomiting

If a child has just vomited and no longer feels nauseated, give small amounts of clear liquids such as water or weak, unsweetened tea. If your child is vomiting but doesn't have any diarrhea, you can also try:

- ginger ale
- diluted cola
- tea
- diluted juice
- sugar water

These liquids provide sugar and won't upset the stomach. However, do not give high-sugar foods to anyone with diarrhea. Always give your child small, frequent sips at first (less than 1 teaspoon), according to Phyllis Stoffman. Don't let the child gulp down an entire 8-ounce glass right after throwing up. If no vomiting follows, you can offer slightly larger amounts very slowly. If the child does vomit again, let her rest and then try a small amount again.

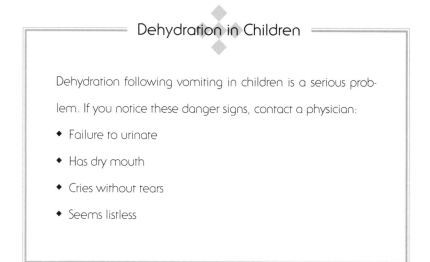

Dehydration in Children

Dehydration following vomiting in children is a serious problem. If you notice these danger signs, contact a physician:

- Failure to urinate
- Has dry mouth
- Cries without tears
- Seems listless

For children under age one, provide prepared electrolyte sugar solutions such as Pedialyte, which is available in drug stores. Recently, frozen Pedialyte popsicles have been developed. These flavored versions of the old standby may be more appealing to young children.

Sugar Water

2 ½ teaspoons granulated sugar
1 quart water at room temperature

Stir the sugar into the water; have your child sip ½ ounce to an ounce every 15 minutes, with the goal being 3 ounces per hour. Don't fill the child up, which could lead to more vomiting, and don't force a child to drink.

What to Feed Next

When one or two hours pass without vomiting and your child is hungry, you can slowly return to solid foods. Give plain, salted crackers followed by small portions of easy-to-digest foods such as scrambled eggs, rice, toast, or pasta. Many doctors advise the BRAT diet — bananas, rice, applesauce, and toast. At the same time, continue to offer clear fluids. Don't allow your child to drink milk until all signs of illness have passed.

If your child is still feeling nauseated or doesn't feel like eating, don't force food. The lack of appetite is probably a sign that the stomach isn't ready to digest food yet.

Back on Track...

If the BRAT diet goes down well, you can begin to offer light protein foods such as boiled eggs, potatoes, baked or boiled chicken, and plain fish. Don't offer high-protein or fatty foods to your child after vomiting; they are too hard to digest.

If your child is breastfeeding, continue. If he is being bottle-fed, dilute regular portions with half water. Return to the complete formula once vomiting has stopped.

Avoid These Herbal Equivalents

By now, most parents have gotten the news that you shouldn't give aspirin to children under age 18 who have a cold, flu, or chickenpox because of the association with a rare but possibly fatal disease known as Reye's Syndrome.

But if you're fond of herbal treatments, you may not realize that some herbs—willow bark, meadowsweet, and wintergreen—are the equivalent of aspirin and should be avoided as well.

Herbal Preparations for the Common Cold: All You Need to Know

HE USE OF HERBS to treat common health conditions has always been an important part of medical care. In fact, the word drug comes from the old Dutch *drogge* (to dry), referring to the practice of drying plants as medicines. About a quarter of all prescription drugs today are derived from trees, shrubs, and herbs. Most drug groups we have today were developed from the plant kingdom, although they may now be produced synthetically.

While most of today's drugs have been derived from herbs, herbs are not equivalent to drugs. Herbs are far less concentrated than the medicines we buy at the drug store. While these milder herbal products are less concentrated, they often contain far more complex combinations of related active ingredients than do prescription medications. For example, the herb digitalis contains more than 30 closely related glycosides, all of which affect the heart in various ways at different speeds. And St. John's wort, an herb noted for its antidepressant action, has many active constituents that combine in ways scientists don't fully understand.

And yet in American society, herbal medicine is not widely accepted. In part, this is because of economics: drug companies don't research herbal remedies because plants can't be patented and why bother to make a pill from a substance that consumers can grow themselves? Moreover, collecting and processing herbs is not as easy as manufacturing synthetic compounds. Finally, most people have simply been conditioned to rely on commercial drugs for quick relief, regardless of potential cost or side effects.

Still, there is evidence that the tendency to avoid herbal and other natural products to treat illnesses is changing, as the race to uncover better treatments continues. There are as many as 500,000 different plants growing on earth today, and only about 5,000 of these have been extensively studied as potential medications. Considering that 121 prescription drugs come from just 90 species of plants, scientists have realized that there may be many more potential cures in the natural world just waiting to be discovered.

How Herbs Work

The chemical constituents of herbs found in the leaf, flower, stem, seed, root, fruit, or bark are the active ingredients that fight disease. Most herbs contain a large variety of natural chemicals, which scientists can extract and purify to provide an "active" compound. For example, the herb foxglove produces digoxin; the Indian herb snakeroot produces reserpine; the opium poppy produces morphine.

However, just because all herbs and plants are natural, it doesn't mean that they are nontoxic. Almost any herb used in excess or for the wrong purposes can cause problems. In fact, some of the most toxic substances in the world are derived from plants. But because plants and herbs travel indirectly to the blood and organs, they tend to work more slowly and less dramatically than commercial medications. This is why some people prefer the quick fix of a modern drug —regardless of the harmful side effects and high cost—to the slower response of an herb or plant.

Herbs may be useful against certain symptoms of the common cold because of a specific chemical in the plant, or because of a complex interaction between different compounds.

Growing Your Own Herbs

Remember that if you're growing herbs to use to treat your cold symptoms, the amount of active compound inside any one herb or plant depends on a host of variables including soil type, water, sun, and nutrients. One plant of a species may have completely different amounts of active compound than its neighbor only a short distance away because it was grown in a slightly different environment, or because it has a slightly different genetic background.

If you are sure you want to grow your own, you can find seeds or plants for most herbs either by mail order or at local nurseries (see Appendix B).

HARVESTING AND DRYING HERBS

If you want to grow and harvest your own herbs, it's important to remember that *when* you gather them affects the potency of each plant, and therefore its ability to treat symptoms. Herbs should be harvested on a dry day when the plant is at the peak of maturity so that the active ingredients will be most concentrated.

Herbs should be dried quickly, away from bright sunshine in a warm (between 70 and 90 degrees F), dry, airy place such as a sunny room or an airing cupboard with the door open. Avoid drying herbs in a damp location or in a garage (gasoline fumes can contaminate the plant). Try to dry your herbs completely within six days, because drying longer may result in discolored or less flavorful plants.

Once the herbs are dry, store them in a dry, dark glass or pottery container with an airtight lid out of direct sunlight. If the herbs are stored in damp areas, they will become moldy. Properly dried, most herbs will keep for up to 18 months.

If you want to harvest and dry your herbs, each part of the plant needs to be handled in a specific way.

BARK

Harvest bark in the fall when the sap is falling so you don't damage the plant. Never remove all the bark from a plant or a band of bark completely from around a tree unless you intend to kill the plant. After you've harvested the bark, wipe off any moss or insects but don't soak in water. Break into smaller pieces of about several inches, spread on a paper-lined tray, and leave to dry.

BULBS

Harvest bulbs after the part of the plant above the ground has wilted. Garlic bulbs should be collected quickly, since they tend to sink into the ground as the leaves wilt and become hard to find.

FLOWERS

Flowers should be harvested just after the morning dew has evaporated, when the buds are fully opened. Small flowers (such as lavender) should be picked before the flowers wither completely.

Cut flower heads from the stems. Remove dirt, grit, or insects and spread on a tray lined with paper or newsprint. When the flower heads are dry, you can store them whole in a dark, airtight container. However, marigolds should not be stored whole; instead, pick off the petals and store individually, throwing away the center of the flower. Lavender should be dried on the stem, upside down in a paper bag or over a tray.

FRUIT

Berries and other fruit should be harvested when just ripe, before the fruit gets too soft to dry well. Spread on paper-lined trays to dry; turn often to ensure even drying. Discard any fruit that begins to mold.

LEAVES

Plants with large leaves can be harvested and dried individually, while plants with smaller leaves should be dried on the stem. Leaves of deciduous herbs should be dried just before they flower; you can gather the evergreen leaves (such as rosemary) all year round.

To dry leaves, tie in small bunches of about 8 to 12 stems and hang upside down to dry. When the leaves are brittle but not so dry that they turn to powder when you touch them, rub them from the stem onto a piece of paper. Pour the dried herbs into an airtight storage container.

ROOTS

Most roots should be harvested in autumn, when the plant has wilted, but before the ground has become too hard. (However, the dandelion should be harvested in spring.) If the root becomes moist and soft after harvesting, discard it because it has absorbed too much moisture from the air.

After harvesting, wash thoroughly to remove soil and dirt. Chop large roots into smaller pieces while fresh. Spread pieces on a paper-lined tray, and dry for 2 or 3 hours in a slightly warm oven (large roots may take 4 to 6 hours). Transfer to a warm, sunny room to finish drying.

SEEDS

The entire seed head should be harvested when the seeds are almost ripe, together with about 5 inches of stalk. Hang away from direct sunlight upside down over a tray lined in paper, or in a paper bag. Seeds will fall off when they are ripe.

Making Your Own Herbal Preparations

Many people enjoy making their own herbal preparations fresh from the garden. Others may want to use plants in a different form — anything from a capsule to a tincture. Some of these can be bought in natural or health food stores, while others you can prepare yourself.

TEAS

The most common way to use herbs to treat cold symptoms is by brewing a cup of tea. Keep in mind, however, that a medicinal tea is not much like a cup of mild-flavored commercial beverage. Medicinal herbal teas are much stronger and often do not taste very good.

You make a cup of herbal medicinal tea by steeping an ounce of dried tops (flowers, leaves, or stems) in a pint of almost-boiling water. Commercially-prepared herbal teas are very mild; they contain only a fraction of the amount of the herbs you're using in each teabag. If you use the actual dried herb to make your medicinal tea, you'll be getting more concentrated oils.

Tips on Brewing Teas, Infusions, and Decoctions

There are a few general recommendations to keep in mind when brewing herbs:

- Don't use aluminum, iron, tin, or other metals to make tea, since the metal can leach into the liquid.

- Use only pure spring water. Avoid chlorinated water and water that might contain other chemicals.

- Boil the water first and then remove it from the heat; don't add herbs into boiling water over the heat.

- Steep with the lid on; if you can smell the aroma of the tea, some of the essential oils are escaping.

- Use 1 ounce of dried herbs to 2 cups of water, or 2 ounces of fresh herbs to 2 cups of water.

In general, you can substitute fresh herbs for dried in a tea recipe, but remember to double the amount of herbs you use. Fresh herbs have more water and therefore, they are much weaker than dried herbs.

INFUSIONS

If you keep on brewing the tea for more than 15 minutes up to an hour or so, it's called an infusion. Infusions aren't usually made by the cup, but in large batches, enough for one day. (One pint should last you through the day.) When you make an infusion, be sure the water is not quite boiling, since vigorously boiling water tends to make the volatile oils evaporate in the steam.

This method should be used for flowers and leafy parts of plants. The standard amount you're going to use should be made fresh each day. You can drink an infusion either hot or cold, depending on your symptoms. For example, if you want to induce sweating or break up a cough or cold, drink the infusion hot.

To make an infusion, pour 1 pint of hot water over ½ to 1 ounce of powdered herb and steep in an enamel, porcelain, or glass pot for 10 to 20 minutes. Then cover with a tight-fitting lid to prevent evaporation, minimizing the loss of active ingredients.

DECOCTIONS

This method is a more vigorous way to extract a plant's active ingredients. It's used for plant parts that won't dissolve quickly in water, such as roots, barks, twigs, and some berries. As with an infusion, a decoction should be made fresh each day, and can be drunk hot or cold.

To make a decoction, soak 1 teaspoon of the dried herb first in an enamel or glass container with 1 cup of pure cold water and then bring it to a boil. (Or you can use 1 ounce of dried herb to 1 pint of water.)

You'll want to simmer the herb for 5 minutes if it is finely shredded, and up to an hour if it is woody. Simmer until the liquid has been reduced by one-third. When the simmering is finished, strain through a nylon sieve into a pitcher or cup while hot. Decoctions should always be strained while hot, although you can drink it hot or cold. Store in a cool place.

MACERATIONS

Some herbs (such as valerian root) work better as a maceration than as either a decoction or an infusion. To make a maceration, pour cold water over the dried herb and leave in a cool place overnight. Strain through a nylon sieve the next morning.

STEAM INHALANTS

If you've got stuffy sinuses or too much mucus, an herbal inhalant may ease the symptoms. Place 1 or 2 tablespoons of dried herbs in a bowl and pour boiling water over it. Lean over the bowl with a towel draped over your head; inhale for as long as you can bear the heat, or until the mixture cools.

Don't go out into the cold for at least a half hour after you've taken the inhalant.

TINCTURES

A tincture is a solution of a concentrated herbal extract made by steeping either dried or fresh herbs with a 25% mixture of alcohol and water. Tinctures can be kept on the shelf for up to two years because the alcohol acts as a preservative.

These preparations are usually made with stronger herbs that might not taste very good, and that usually aren't drunk as an herbal tea. You can use any part of the plant, but each tincture should be made with individual herbs. Once the tincture is made, you can then combine it with a tincture made from a different plant.

Commercial tinctures use ethyl alcohol, but you can use diluted spirits such as vodka if you make it yourself at home. Vodka is considered the best choice since it has few additives; use rum to disguise the taste of unpleasant-tasting herbs.

To make a tincture, combine 4 ounces of powdered or cut herb with 1 pint of alcohol (vodka, brandy, gin, or rum) or vinegar in a large jar. The plant material should be covered by the alcohol. Seal the jar and store in a cool place for 2 weeks; shake every day. After the herbs settle to the bottom, pour off the tincture and strain out the powder through cheesecloth. Pour the strained liquid into clean, dark glass bottles. Use a funnel, if necessary.

❖❖CAUTION: Don't use industrial alcohol, methylated spirits (methyl alcohol), or rubbing alcohol (isopropyl alcohol) in tinctures. All of these types of alcohol are extremely toxic.

EXTRACTS

An extract is made by combining 4 ounces of dried herbs (or 8 ounces of fresh herbs) into a jar with 1 pint of vinegar, alcohol, or massage oil. Shake the bottle once or twice a day for 4 days if the herbs are powdered, and 2 weeks if the herbs are fresh. The following extracts are especially good for treating the common cold:

Catnip and fennel extract: Treats nausea, fevers, headaches, and restlessness.

Garlic oil: Good for respiratory infections.

Goldenseal root: An excellent choice for general cold symptoms, especially a runny nose and sneezing.

CREAMS

A cream is a mixture of fat or oil with water that will blend in with the skin. Creams can easily be made using an emulsifying ointment (available from a drugstore), which is a mixture of oils and waxes that blend with water.

Homemade creams will last for a few months; to preserve them even longer, store the cream in the refrigerator, or add a few drops of benzoin tincture as a preservative. Remember that creams made from organic oils and fat deteriorate more quickly.

To make a cream, melt the fat and water in a bowl over boiling water; add the herbs and heat on low for 3 hours. Place a cheesecloth around another bowl and strain the mixture. Stir constantly until cold, and then place in small jars.

OINTMENTS

An ointment is a combination of herbs in an oil base (preferably made from natural sources instead of from petroleum products). Ointments contain only oils or fats—no water. Unlike creams, ointments don't blend in with the skin; instead, they form a layer over the skin.

To make an ointment, melt the wax or jelly in a bowl over a pan of boiling water and stir in 1 or 2 heaping tablespoons of the herb. Heat for about 2 hours until the herbs are crisp. Pour the mixture into a cheesecloth fitted over a jar and tied with string or a rubber band. While the mixture is still hot, put on rubber gloves and untie the cheesecloth; holding the cheesecloth over the jar, squeeze the mixture through the cheesecloth into the jar. Quickly pour the strained mixture while still warm into clean glass storage jars.

OILS

You can extract active plant ingredients in oil if they aren't going to be taken internally. Infused oils will last for up to a year if you store them in a dark, cool place, but smaller amounts made fresh may be more potent. There are two methods for oil infusions: cold and hot. Hot infusions are suitable for herbs such as chickweed or rosemary; cold infusions work well with marigold or St. John's wort.

Alternatively, you can gently heat the oil and herbs in a double boiler for 3 hours; strain through a cheesecloth into a clean, airtight bottle. You can add a small amount of vitamin E to help preserve the preparation. Oils are usually made from a strong-smelling herb such as peppermint, eucalyptus, or spearmint.

A cold infusion begins by pounding fresh herbs and then packing them into a large jar and covering it completely with olive or sesame oil, then leaving it in a warm place for about 4 days.

You can make a cream or ointment from infused oil by thickening the hot or cold infused oil with beeswax and water-free lanolin. For a cream, melt equal parts of beeswax with water-free lanolin and add 5 tablespoons of infused oil and ¼ cup herbal tincture. Strain and store in clean, dark glass jars while still warm; allow to cool.

✦✦CAUTION: Never ingest any kind of herbal oil. Many herbs that are safe when used as infusions are toxic when highly concentrated in the form of an essential oil.

COMPRESSES

Some herbs work best by being applied on the skin, either in a compress or a poultice, especially the "hot" or "spicy" herbs such as mustard, cayenne, and ginger, or the "cooling" herbs, such as slippery elm, borage, and aloe. All of these external remedies should be used in a warm room to keep you feeling comfortable.

A compress is simply a cloth pad soaked in a hot herbal extract, used when herbs are too strong to be taken internally. They are prepared with boiling water so that the herb is combined with heat to ease swelling, pain, cold, or the flu. It also can stimulate the flow of blood in the body. A cold compress can be used to ease a headache.

✦✦CAUTION: To avoid getting burned, be sure that the liquid is not hotter than 180 degress F, and make sure that you wring out the towel or pad you're using thoroughly.

Infusions, decoctions and tinctures (diluted with water) all can be used for a compress. For a pad, you can choose soft cotton or linen, a cotton ball, or surgical sterile gauze.

To make an herbal compress, add 1 or 2 tablespoons of the herb to 1 cup of hot water. Strain the liquid and then dip in a cotton pad or sterile gauze. Squeeze out excess liquid and place on the affected area while still warm, covering it with a piece of woolen material. Change the compress when it cools down or dries out.

Remove the compress if your skin becomes red, or if you feel uncomfortable.

POULTICES

A poultice is similar to a compress, but this time the whole herb is used instead of a liquid extract; the warm herb is applied directly to the skin. Poultices are usually applied when they are hot, although cold fresh leaves may also work.

Fresh herbs can be chopped in a food processor for a few seconds, or boiled in water for 2 to 5 minutes. Dried herbs can be decocted; powders can be mixed with a little water to make a paste. Moisten the powdered herb with hot water, apple cider vinegar, or herbal tea.

To draw out a fever, try squeezing the water from tofu and mash with flour and about 5 percent fresh grated gingerroot. Onion poultices are especially useful for sore throats. (When used as a poultice, chop and heat the onions.)

❖❖❖CAUTION: Don't use stronger herbs such as cayenne or mustard because direct contact with the skin could cause a burn. Use these herbs in a plaster instead.

PLASTERS

A plaster is similar to a compress or poultice, except that the herbs or herb paste is applied within the folds of muslin or cheesecloth and applied to the skin. Stronger herbs (cayenne or mustard, for example) are best used as a plaster so they don't directly contact the skin.

POWDERS/CAPSULES

You can also take an herb as a powder that is stirred into water or sprinkled on food, or you can make the herbs into a capsule if they don't taste very good. Capsules are also a good choice if you're on the go and need to take your herbs on the run.

The first pills were not manufactured by drug companies, but by the Shaker herbalists who found that sending bulk herbs through the mail was difficult.

It's a good idea to use commercially-prepared powders, which you can buy from health food suppliers. If you try to grind the herbs yourself, you will likely generate heat which can cause chemical changes in the herb. You can buy two-part gelatin or vegetarian capsule cases from health food suppliers.

If you want to try making a powder, mash fresh plant parts into fine particles so the herb can be taken in a capsule, water, herb tea, or sprinkled on food.

To fill capsules, pour the powdered herb into a saucer, separate the two halves of a capsule case, and slide them together through the powder, scooping as you go. Fit the two ends of the capsule together and store in a dark glass jar in a cool place.

SYRUPS

A syrup is a good way to treat a cough, congestion, or a sore throat, since it coats the throat and keeps the herb in contact with the painful part of the body. Herbal syrups are a simple, effective way to preserve the healing quality of herbs.

To make a syrup, add about 2 ounces of dried herb to a quart of water, and gently boil down to 1 pint. Add 2 ounces of honey or glycerine while still warm. Licorice or wild cherry bark are often used as flavorings. Other good herbs to choose include anise seed, fennel seed, or Irish moss. If you use fresh fruit, leaves, or roots to make a syrup, double the amount of herbs you include. Herbal syrups should be stored in the refrigerator.

JUICES

You can make herb juices using a food processor or juicer. Squeeze the pulp through a nylon sieve or cheesecloth to obtain the juice. Keep in mind, however, that you'll need large amounts of fresh herb to get enough juice.

Are Herbs Safe?

While some people worry that taking herbs seems to be riskier than taking drugs, the American Association of Poison Control Centers found this not to be the case. In one recent two-year study, the Association found that medications caused 974 deaths and 6,978 major nonfatal poisonings; plants caused 3 deaths and 53 major poisonings. Indeed, some of the most toxic plants are not herbs at all, but ornamental varieties, such as holly, jade, philodendron, and dieffenbachia.

This doesn't mean that herbs won't hurt if you if ingest too much or don't understand what you are taking. In recent years, some herbs that had been considered safe—such as comfrey—have, in fact, been found to be toxic and, of course, almost any herb can cause an allergic reaction in some people.

In general, most herbal remedies should probably not be given to children under age 2; herbs should be used in smaller amounts for youngsters under age 16 and adults over age 65. Anyone with a chronic condition should consult a physician before using any natural remedy to ease the symptoms of the common cold.

GETTING THE RIGHT DOSE

If you get your herbs from a commercial source, you'll find that companies standardize certain doses so that you know exactly how much of the active ingredient you're getting. It is much more difficult to know exactly what the dose is when you buy bulk herbs or if you grow your own. Fortunately, the active constituents in herbs tend to be far less potent than commercial drug preparations, so slight variations may not be crucial.

CONSULTING AN HERBALIST

While you can use these herbs to treat the common cold, a persistent problem may require some advice from a qualified herbalist. Some herbalists prescribe specific herbal remedies to ease your symptoms, while others may focus on more holistic treatments that suggest lifestyle changes as well. Your herbalist may also give you advice about what foods to eat or avoid, relaxation techniques, and other natural treatments.

The first consultation with an herbalist usually takes about an hour; follow-up visits may only last 20 minutes or so.

Experts in the science of herbs may use approaches based on an Asian approach (Chinese medicine or the Indian system of Ayurveda), or they may be naturopathic physicians. There are many organizations that will help you find qualified health providers in herbal medicine; addresses for many of these are found in Appendix A at the end of this book.

CHINESE MEDICINE

Traditional Chinese medicine emphasizes the restoration of harmony, as expressed in the five elements (fire, earth, metal, water, and wood) and two complementary forces — the yin and the yang. Herbs are an important part of this balance.

Your first visit to a practitioner will probably cost between $60 and $110; follow-up visits range from about $30 to $80. Thirty-six states license Chinese medicine practitioners, but their requirements vary. In states that don't license these practitioners, practice is limited to physicians with an M.D. or D.O. (doctor of osteopathy).

There are about 17,000 traditional Chinese medicine practitioners now certified and licensed to practice in the United States. Practitioners should have completed at least a two-year science program and a three- or four-year program specializing in Chinese medicine. Within the United States, you're most likely to find a traditional Chinese medicine practitioner in California, Oregon, Washington, Florida, New Mexico, New York, or Colorado. To find a practitioner near you, you can contact the American Association of Oriental Medicine at (610) 266-1433 for a national listing of practitioners.

AYURVEDA

To a much greater degree than Chinese medicine, Ayurvedic medicine focuses on a healthy lifestyle as the source of disease prevention and cure. Rooted in the ancient Indian culture, Ayurveda is the oldest recorded healing therapy still used today. The medicines and philosophies of Ayurveda have been described in texts dating back several thousand years. The term Ayurveda is Sanskrit for the science (or knowledge) of life. Practitioners recognize five elements: ether, fire, water, air, and earth; Ayurvedic physicians try to balance the elements of air or wind, fire or bile, and water or phlegm, and use herbs in this effort. An Ayurvedic physician would be interested in what and when you eat, where you live, who your friends are, your environment and activity level, sleep and recreation patterns, and so on. The tradition is based on the belief that each person is born with a predominant dosha or combination of doshas, which govern bodily functions and personality. When your doshas are in balance, you're healthy; if they are unbalanced, you might catch a cold. An Ayurvedic physician will tell you that you can't expect a natural remedy to ease your cold symptoms if you aren't living in harmony with nature.

The average cost of an initial visit may range from $100 to $150, depending on the part of the country in which you live. At present, Ayurvedic practitioners aren't covered by health insurance.

There are a few Ayurvedic clinics in this country, which hire one or more Ayurvedic physicians. More than 200 physicians have trained through the American Association of Ayurvedic Medicine, and use Ayurveda in their medical practice. You'll be most likely to find a practitioner on either the East or West coast, although the tradition is becoming more popular in other parts of the country.

Ayurveda has no legal status in the United States, so practitioners aren't licensed or certified. The U.S. Food and Drug Administration restricts the use of some of the herbs that are commonly used by Ayurvedic practitioners in India. For more information, contact the Chopra Center for Well Being at (619) 551-7119 or the Ayurvedic Institute at (505) 291-9698.

NATUROPATHY

Naturopathic medicine can treat the symptoms of the common cold by using the body's inborn ability to heal itself with a variety of alternative methods based on your particular needs. Naturopathic doctors stress the importance of healing the person, not the disease. Methods may include nutrition counseling, herbal medicine, homeopathy, acupuncture, hydrotherapy, physical medicine, counseling, and lifestyle moderation. Seven states license naturopathic physicians: Alaska, Arizona, Connecticut, Hawaii, Montana, Oregon, and Washington, and seven other states are considering their own licensing provisions. Five Canadian provinces also license naturopaths: Alberta, British Columbia, Manitoba, Ontario, and Saskatchewan.

Accredited colleges of naturopathic medicine include Bastyr University in Seattle, Washington; National College of Naturopathic Medicine in Portland, Oregon; Southwest College in Scottsdale, Arizona; and Canadian College of Naturopathic Medicine in Etobicoke, Ontario.

Unfortunately, at this point in time, only a few insurance companies will reimburse you for the services of a naturopathic physician.

Additional Resources for Natural Healing

Organizations and Associations

Acupressure Institute of America
1533 Shattuck Ave.
Berkeley, CA 94709
This institute offers several acupuncture training programs.

Alliance Foundation for Alternative Medicine
PO Box 59
Liberty Lake, WA 99010
(509) 255-9246
An organization that is active in education, politics, and collecting clinical data on the effectiveness of alternative medicine. The Alliance maintains a worldwide network of political advocates who promote the cause of alternative therapy. They offer material on current research, and they maintain lists of alternative health care practitioners. They also offer an 8-page newsletter.

American Academy of Medical Acupuncture
5820 Wilshire Blvd., Suite 500
Los Angeles, CA 90036
(800) 521-2262 Physican referral line
Leave your name and address for a list of medical doctors who practice acupuncture in your area.

American Aromatherapy Association
PO Box 3679
South Pasadena, CA 91301
(818) 457-1742
A professional organization of aromatherapists that helps to establish standards and provide certification and training to its members. The Association maintains a directory of members and will help you locate a professional aromatherapist in your area.

American Association of Acupuncture and Oriental Medicine
4101 Lake Boone Trail, Suite 201
Raleigh, NC 27607
(919) 787-5181
This national professional organization of acupuncturists includes those who meet acceptable standards of competency. The group can provide you with the names and locations of members in your area.

American Association of Naturopathic Physicians
2366 Eastlake Ave., Suite 322
Seattle, WA 98102
(206) 323-7610
This group can provide you with names of licensed naturopathic physicians in your area.

American Botanical Council
PO Box 201660
Austin, TX 78720
(512) 331-8868
http://www.herbalgram.org
Publishes HerbalGram, a magazine that answers questions about herbs, and conducts herbal research.

American Herb Association
PO Box 353
Rescue, CA 95672
(916) 626-5046
This group promotes herbal education and seeks to increase the use of herbs and herbal products. The group publishes several herbal source directories of seeds, plants, and other items.

American Herbalists Guild
PO Box 746555
Arvada, CO 80006
(303) 423-8800
Provides referrals to qualified herbalists and herbal education programs.

American Holistic Medical Association
4101 Lake Boone Trail, Suite 201
Raleigh, NC 27607
(919) 787-5181
For a fee, this group can provide referrals. They publish a bimonthly magazine, several other publications, and guidelines for nutrition and fitness. They also sponsor conferences on holistic medicine for the holistic professional.

American Holistic Nurses' Association
4101 Lake Boone Trail, Suite 201
Raleigh, NC 27607
(919) 787-5181
A professional nursing organization that believes that the major purpose of nursing is to help other professionals toward the health of the patient. The Association defines health as the harmonious balance of mind, body, and spirit—not the relief of symptoms defined in a medical textbook. Membership is open only to professional nurses.

American Massage Therapy Association

820 Davis St., Suite 1000

Evanston, IL 60201

This association provides referrals of certified massage therapists and certified massage schools in your area.

American School of Ayurvedic Sciences

10025 NE 4th St.

Bellevue, WA 98004

(206) 453-8022

This college provides medical training for physicians and health care practitioners as well as individual courses for lay students. Dr. Virender Sodhi's Ayurvedic, Naturopathic Medical Clinic is located at this same address.

Association of Holistic Healing Centers

2100 Mediterranean Ave., Suite 40

Virginia Beach, VA 23451

(804) 498-2598

This professional organization of individuals, groups, and centers involved in healing strives to educate, sponsor conferences and workshops, and create prototype healing centers. Membership is open to anyone interested or involved in the healing arts. A directory of members is available to health care consumers interested in a referral.

Association of Health Practitioners

PO Box 5007

Durango, CO 81301

(303) 259-1091

A professional group of dentists and physicians who provide alternative therapies and oppose the use of toxic materials or those with the potential of being toxic. They also offer referrals to members in your area.

Biofeedback Certification Institute of America

10200 West 44th Ave., Suite 304

Wheat Ridge, CO 80033

Write for a list of certified biofeedback therapists in your area.

College of Maharishi Ayurveda Medical Center

PO Box 282

Fairfield, IA 52556

(515) 472-5866

Provides referrals to health centers that offer treatment or prevention for a broad range of illnesses. The center also trains practitioners and provides information to the public.

Herbal Research Foundation

1007 Pearl St., #200

Boulder, CO 80302

800-748-2617; (303) 449-2265

Provides free information packets on herbs and health conditions, and provides a list of schools of herbal medicine.

Homeopathic Academy of Naturopathic Physicians

14653 Graves Rd.

Mulino, OR 97042

(503) 829-7326

A professional organization of naturopaths (NDs) who use classical homeopathy as one of their treatment modalities. The organization publishes a journal (Simillimum), and offers a referral list of naturopaths who use classical homeopathy in their practice.

Homeopathic Educational Services

2124 Kittredge St.

Berkeley, CA 94704

(415) 649-0294

Provides general information in books, audio tapes, software, and kits. They also offer prepared homeopathic medicines for minor ailments.

International Foundation for Homeopathy
2366 Eastlake Ave. East, Suite 301
Seattle, WA 98102
A group that provides educational courses for professionals and the general public. Offers referrals to homeopathic health professionals.

National Association for Holistic Aromatherapy
PO Box 17622
Boulder, CO 80308
(303) 258-3791
An organization of professional aromatherapists trained by the London School of Aromatherapy; all are certified by and are members of the International Federation of Aromatherapists. A nonprofessional member can receive the quarterly newsletter, Scentsitivity. The Association also maintains a referral list and will help you locate an aromatherapist in your area.

National Center for Homeopathy
801 N. Fairfax, Suite 306
Alexandria, VA 22314
Provides a referral list of practicing homeopaths and related information. Gives courses for lay students and professionals, and organizes study groups around the country.

National Commission for the Certification of Acupuncturists
1424 16th St. NW
Washington, DC 20036
More than 3,000 acupuncturists have been certified in the U.S. For a list of certified acupuncturists in your state, send a $3 check or money order to cover postage and handling to:

National Commission for the Certification of Acupuncturists
P.O. Box 9797
Washington, DC 20090

World Research Foundation
15300 Ventura Blvd., Suite 405
Sherman Oaks, CA 91403
(818) 907-5483
This group's main purpose is to gather and make available information on health and the environment from around the world. It provides information on alternative health care and preventive techniques, and offers lectures, seminars, publications, tapes, and videos on new alternative therapies, as well as library searches from a collection of more than 500 journals from 100 countries and 100,000 books. There is also computer access to more than 500 databases of traditional pharmaceutical and surgical treatments. A minimum donation entitles you to receive the Foundation's quarterly publication, World Research Journal.

Publications

Alternatives for the Health Conscious Individual
Mountain Home Publishing
PO Box 829
Ingram, TX 78025
(512) 367-4492
Eight-page newsletter that provides information on prevention and alternative treatments for a wide range of diseases.
Monthly. $39 per year

American Herb Quarterly Newsletter
American Herb Association
PO Box 353
Rescue, CA 95672

(916) 626-5046
Publication with short, well-researched articles on a variety of
herbal health issues.
Quarterly. $20 per year.

Beginnings
A publication of the American Holistic Nurses' Association, (see
page 173) this magazine includes news of holistic nursing, a calen-
dar of upcoming events, and other related features.
Monthly. $16 per year.

Bio-Research for Global Evolution
PO Box 3427
Eugene, OR 97403
(503) 345-9855
This four page newsletter places a special emphasis on nutrition,
natural approaches to disease, regenerative therapy, and anti-stress
methodologies. Each issue is devoted to a single topic. Back issues,
reprints, and books are also available.
Monthly. $20 per year.

Common Scents
American Aromatherapy Association
PO Box 3679
South Pasadena, CA 91301
(818) 457-1742
Journal that includes articles on both technical information and
business matters relating to the profession.
Quarterly. $30 a year.

Health World
1477 Rollins Rd.
Burlingame, CA 94010
(415) 343-1637

This full-color publication features advice on health from an alternative viewpoint, including vitamins, nutrition, health food, chiropractic, homeopathy, and Chinese medicine. Regular monthly columns provide updated information; all articles are scholarly but free of jargon, and are usually written by scientists rather than journalists.
Bimonthly. $10.50 per year.

HerbalGram

A joint publication of the American Botanical Council and the Herb Research Foundation, this newsletter provides book reviews and roundups of current trends.
Quarterly. $25 per year.
For more information: (512) 331-8868

The Herb Companion

A magazine that discusses culinary and medicinal uses of herbs. The Herb Research Foundation and the American Herbalists Guild provide a "Herbs for Health" section in each issue.
Bimonthly. $24 per year.
For more information: (800) 645-3675

Holistic Medicine

This 30-page journal of the American Holistic Medical Association provides articles directed toward the professional, including clinical case studies, in-depth information on prevention and treatment, book reviews, news, and upcoming events.
Bimonthly. $25 (includes membership in the AHMA)

International Journal of Aromatherapy

Essential Imports
401 Neptune Ave., Suite B
Encinitas, CA 92024
(619) 944-8481

The only scientifically-based medical journal on the subject, published by the Tisserand Institute of Great Britain. All articles are technical, and each subject is covered in depth. Most have references and citations from professional literature.
Quarterly. $50 per year.

Journal of Alternative and Complementary Medicine
Argus Health Publications
Manner House
53A High St.
Bag Shot, Surrey, GU 19 5AH
United Kingdom
0235-353535
JACM is the foremost British publication devoted exclusively to alternative and complementary medicine, written for health care professionals and interested individuals. It is available only through subscription from its United Kingdom publishers.

Journal of Naturopathic Medicine
Journal Management Group, Inc.
10 Morgan Ave.
Norwalk, CT 06851
(203) 661-7375
Journal designed for health care professionals seeking rigorous, scientific information on holistic treatments for common and chronic ailments.
Quarterly. $65 per year.

Medical Herbalism:
A Clinical Newsletter for the Herbal Practitioner
A 12-page newsletter with research data focusing on the use of herbs as medicine.
Quarterly. $36 per year.
For more information: (303) 541-9552.

Natural Health Magazine
PO Box 7440
Red Oak, IA 51591
Consumer magazine dedicated to an exploration of alternative
health possibilities.
Bimonthly. $24 per year

Scentsitivity
National Association for Holistic Aromatherapy
PO Box 17622
Boulder, CO 80308
(303) 258-3791
A 12-page publication on aromatherapy, with articles aimed at a
lay audience.
Quarterly. $35 per year

Suppliers of Hard-to-Find Herbs and Seeds

If you want to grow some of your own plants and herbs for the natural remedies provided in this book, you can order seeds from the following companies. These companies are particularly helpful when you are trying to grow plants and herbs that are not always readily available.

Burpee and Company
300 Park Avenue
Warminster, PA 18991
Phone: (800) 888-1447
Fax: (800) 487-5530

Johnny's Selected Seeds
Foss Hill Road
Albion, ME 04910-9731
Phone: (207) 437-4301
Fax: (207) 437-2165

Nichols Garden Nursery
1190 North Pacific Highway
Albany, OR 97321-4580
Phone: (541) 928-9280

Seeds Blum
HC 33, Idaho City Stage
Boise, ID 83706
Phone: (800) 742-1423
Fax: (208) 333-5658

Seeds of Change
1364 Rufina Circle #5
Santa Fe, NM 87501
Phone: (505) 438-8080
Fax: (505) 438-7052

Sheperd's Garden Seeds
30 Irene Street
Torrington, CT 06790
Phone: (203) 482-3638
Fax: (203) 482-0532

*Sheperd's also has operators
taking orders in California:*

Phone: (408) 335-6910
Fax: (408) 335-2080

Smith and Hawken
Two Arbor Lane
P.O. Box 6900
Florence, KY 41022-6900
Phone: (800) 776-3336
Fax: (606) 727-1166
To order a catalogue:
(800) 981-9888

Southern Exposure
Seed Exchange
P.O. Box 170
Earlysville, VA 22936
Phone: (804) 973-4703
Fax: (804) 973-8717

Territorial Seed Company
P.O. Box 157
Cottage Grove, OR 97424
Phone: (541) 942-9547
Fax: (888) 657-3131

Vermont Bean Seed
Company
Garden Lane
Fairhaven, VT 05743
Phone: (802) 273-3400

Following is a list of suppliers of fresh herbs, especially those that might be hard to find:

Creation Gardens
609 East Main Street
Louisville, KY 40403
Phone: (502) 587-9012
(Also carries almost all
varieties of mushrooms)

Dean & DeLuca
560 Broadway
New York, NY 10012
Phone: (800) 221-7714
(212) 431-1691

Frieda's Finest
4465 Corporate Center Drive
Los Alamitos, CA 90720
Phone: (800) 421-9744
(714) 826-6100

Herb Time Farms
P.O. Box 2862
San Francisco, CA 94083
Phone: (415) 952-4372

Quail Mountain Herbs
P.O. Box 1049
Watsonville, CA 95077-1049
Phone: (408) 722-8456
Fax: (408) 722-9472

References

Akerele, O. "WHO Guidelines for the Assessment of Herbal Medicines." Fitoterapia 62 (1992) 99-110; summarized in HerbalGram 28 (1993) :13-20.

Balch, James and Balch, Phyllis. *Prescription for Nutritional Healing*. New Hyde Park, NY: Avery Publishing Group, 1996.

Beinfeld, Harriet and Korngold, Efrem, *Between Heaven and Earth: A Guide to Chinese Medicine*. New York: Ballantine Books, 1991.

Benedict, Martha. "Holistic Approaches to Colds and Flu." *Body Mind Spirit*. February/March 1995, 14: 16-17.

Bensky, Dan and Gamble, Andrew. *Chinese Herbal Medicine Materia Medica*. Seattle: Eastland Press, 1986.

Bisset, N.G. (ed.). *Herbal Drugs and Phytopharmaceuticals*. Stuttgart: Medpharm Scientific, 1994.

Blakeslee, Sandra. "Is Ordinary Baker's Yeast Old Secret to Curing Common Cold?" *The New York Times*, Nov. 22, 1994.

Brody, Jane. "Colds and Flu." *Woman's Day*. Nov. 1, 1995, 74-77.

___. *Jane Brody's Cold and Flu Fighter*. New York: W.W. Norton, 1995.

___. "Test Your Antibiotics IQ." *The New York Times*. March 13, 1996; NYT website.

Blumenthal, Mark. "Echinacea Highlighted as Cold and Flu Remedy." HerbalGram 29 (1993): 8-9.

Burton Goldberg Group. *Alternative Medicine, the Definitive Guide*. Fife, WA: Future Medicine Publishing, 1994.

Carey, Sarah. "Don't Be Quick to Pick Cough Syrup Just Because It's Thick." *University of Florida Health Newsnet*, Feb. 14, 1997.

Carroll, David. *The Complete Book of Natural Medicines*. New York: Summit, 1980.

Carstensen, E.J. "Colds: How to Know...What to Do...When." The Medical Reporter website. Oct. 1, 1996.

Casano, Peter J. "The Common Cold," website brochure.

Cassidy, Catherine (ed.). "299 Natural Cures." In *Healing Herbs*. Emmaus, PA: Rodale Press, 1996.

Castleman, Michael. "New Cold and Flu Strategies." *Family Circle.* Jan. 11, 1994, 69-72.

——. "Uncommon Remedies." *Natural Health.* November-December 1994, 90-93; 126-129.

——. "The Hazards of Over-the-Counter Cold Remedies." *Natural Health.* November-December 1994, 91.

——. "Get Relief from Cold Symptoms with Acupressure." *Natural Health.* November-December 1994, 92.

——. *Cold Cures.* New York: Fawcett, 1987.

——. "Eucalyptus." *The Herb Quarterly.* Winter 1991: 17-20.

——. *The Healing Herbs.* Emmaus, PA: Rodale Press, 1991.

Chopra, Deepak. *Perfect Health.* New York: Harmony Books, 1990.

Consumer Guide editors. "11 Tips for Fighting the Cold War." In *Home Remedies Handbook.* Lincolnwood, IL: Publications International, 1993.

Consumer Reports editors. "Finding the Right Cold Medicine." Consumer's Union website, Jan. 1996.

Cooper, Glenda and Arthur, Charles. "Cure for the Common Cold — or Not?" *The Independent* (London); The New York Times Syndicate website, June 18, 1996.

Curtis, F.C. "Colds and Coughs." In *Old Tamaracks' Collection.* Hammond, Ind: Hammond Book Co, 167-169.

Demargaux, N. *Phytotherapy: A Practical Handbook of Herbal Medicine.* Surrey, UK: Herbal Health Publishers, LTD., 1989.

De Smet, P.A. "Should Herbal Medicine-like Products be Licensed as Medicines?" *British Medical Journal* 310, 1995: 1023-1027.

Duke, James A. "Medical Botany: Major Medicinal Plants." Website http://www.inform/umd.edu/EdRes/Colleges/LFSC/life-sciences.plant_biology/duke/li.

Duncan, Alice Likowski. *Your Healthy Child.* Los Angeles: Jeremy Tarcher, 1991.

East-West editors. "A Capsule Look at the New Herbs." *East West.* August 1988: 33.

Elmore, Durr. "Allium Cepa: The Common Red Onion." *Resonance.* May-June 1992: 9-11.

Engle, Janet P. "Counseling on Colds." *American Druggist* (Jan. 1995) 211:36-37.

Feder, David, "Teatime Remedies." *Better Homes and Gardens*.
April 1997: 88.

Foreman, Judy. "The Rush is on to Echinacea." *The Boston Globe*.
March 18,1997; internet reprint.

Foster, Steven and Yue Chongzi. *Herbal Emissaries: Bringing Chinese Herbs to the West*. Rochester, NY: Healing Arts Press, 1992.

Gagnon, Daniel. "Herbal Care for Colds and Flu." *Herbs for Health*. 1,2 (Sept.-Oct. 1996): 34-39.

Gannon, Kathi. "The Many Faces of the Common Cold: What to Do."
Drug Topics 138 (March 7, 1994) :35.

Griffith, H. Winter. "Common Cold." In *Complete Guide to Symptoms, Illness, and Surgery*. New York: Putnam Berkeley Group, 1995.

Haas, Elson. *Staying Healthy with Nutrition*. Berkeley: Celestial Arts, 1992.

Hageman, Sharon L.. "Wondrous Wintergreen." *The Herb Quarterly*.
Winter 1993: 52-53.

Hahn, G. "Hypericum Perforatum — A Medicinal Herb Used in
Antiquity and Still of Interest Today." *Journal of Naturopathic
Medicine* 3:1 (1992), 94-96.

Hamlin, Suzanne. "Take 2 Bowls of Garlic Pasta, Then Call Me in the
Morning." *The New York Times*. 144 (Jan.25, 1995): C1.

Harris, Lloyd J. *The Book of Garlic*. Reading, MA: Addison Wesley
Publishing Co.

HealthFacts editors. "Cold Remedies: Which Ones Provide Relief?"
HealthFacts 19 (Nov. 1994) :1-5.

HealthGate editors. "Common Cold." In *Complete Guide to Symptoms, Illness & Surgery*. HealthGate website.

Heller, Linda. "How Stuff for a Stuffy Nose." *Health*. Feb.-March 1992:
22-26.

Herbs for Health editors. "The Latest on Vitamin C, Zinc and the
Common Cold." *Herbs for Health*. September/October 1997: 65.

Hoffmann, D. *The New Holistic Herbal*. Rockport, ME: Element Books,
1992.

Huang, Kee Chang. *The Pharmacology of Chinese Herbs*. Boca Raton,
FL: CRC, 1993.

Hudson, J.B., Lopez-Bazzocchi, I. and Towers, G. "Antiviral Activities
of Hypericin." *Antiviral Research* 15:2 (1991) :101-112.

Hutchens, A. *A Handbook of Native American Herbs*. Boston: Shambhala,
1992.

Iconis, Rosemary. "When a Cold or Flu Virus Gets Past Our Line of Defense." *Current Health* 21 (Feb. 1995) :13-15.

Kemper, Kathi. *The Holistic Pediatrician: A Parent's Comprehensive Guide to Safe and Effective Therapies for the 25 Most Common Childhood Ailments.* New York: Harper Perennial, 1996.

Khoe, Willem H. "Acupuncture in the Treatment of Infectious Diseases." *American Journal of Acupuncture* 4/3 (July-Sept. 1976) :245-251.

Kirchheimer and the editors of Prevention. *The Doctors' Book of Home Remedies II.* New York: Bantam, 1995.

Kruzel, Tom. "Will We Ever Find a Cure for the Common Cold?" Health-world, American Association of Naturopathic Physicians website.

Lad, Vasant. *Ayurveda: The Science of Self-Healing.* Wilmot, CA: Lotus Light Press, 1984.

Lampert, Leslie. "The Cold War." *Ladies Home Journal.* Feb. 1995, 156.

Lavie, G., et.al. "Hypericin as an Inactivator of Infectious Viruses in Blood Components." *Transfusion* 35:5 (1995) 392-400.

Lee, Kate and Carlin, Peter. "Should You Try Mind-body Medicine?" *Health.* January/February 1997, 76-77

Lee, Paul A. "Echinacea." *Total Health.* August 1990, 50-51.

Long, Patricia. "Herbal Remedies Really Can Fight Off Colds, Headaches and Other Ills—If You Know How to Use Them Safely." *Health.* 1995 website reprint.

Mars, B. "An Herbalist's Approach." *Herbs for Health.* Nov./Dec. 1996, 53.

Mayell, Mark. "50 Do-it-yourself Remedies." *Natural Health.* April 1997,115-129;178-184.

——. *Off-The-Shelf Natural Health.* New York: Bantam Books, 1995.

McCaleb, "Straight Talk on Herbs." *Natural Health.* March-April 1997, 42-44.

Moore, Michael. *Medicinal Plants of the Mountain West.* Santa Fe, NM: Museum of New Mexico Press, 1979.

——. *Medicinal Plants of the Pacific West.* Santa Fe, NM: Red Crane Books, 1993.

Mossad, Sherif B. et.al. "Common Cold: Steps to a Cure." *Annals of Internal Medicine* 125 (July 1996) 89-97; 142-144.

Mott, Peggy. "The 'Cold' Facts About Upper Respiratory Infections." University of Wisconsin-Madison website, July 1994.

Mowrey, D.B. *The Scientific Validation of Herbal Medicine.* New Canaan, CT: Keats Publishing, 1986.

Murray, Michael T. "Common Cold." In An *Encyclopedia of Natural Medicine*. Rocklin, CA: Prima Publishing.

Natural Health editors. "Cold Advice." *Natural Health*. September/October 1994, 22.

Newscenter 4 . "Uncommon Remedies for the Common Cold." Website, 1996.

Nordenberg, Tamar. "Colds and Flu." *FDA Consumer*. October 1996: 15-18.

Norton, Clark. "The Purple Coneflower's Comeback." *Health* 6 (September 1992) :26-27.

Ody, P. *The Complete Medicinal Herbal*. London: Dorling Kindersley, 1993.

Pizzorno, Lara. "What's In Your Medicine Cabinet?" *Delicious!* Sept. 1994, 36-37.

Poppy, John. "How to Make Colds Less Common." *Men's Health*. Jan.-Feb. 1994, 30-31.

Radetsky, Peter. "Cold Front: What's New and What Works." *American Health*. Oct. 1993, 56-62.

Raichlen, Steven. "Curing the Common Cold." *L.A. Times*. March 14, 1996, H-23.

Salaman, Maureen Kennedy. "The Common Cold." *Health Freedom News*. March-April 1988, 67.

Saloman, Jennifer. "Spotlight on Herbs." *Natural Health*. May-June 1997, 22.

Savard, Marie. "Get Back in the Pink." *Woman's Day*. Aug. 6, 1996, 40.

Schaaf, Rachelle. "Are Antibiotics Used Too Early?" *Parents*, April 1997, 39.

Schechter, Steve. "Protect Your Family from Colds and Flu." *Delicious!* Sept. 1994, 42-43.

Shapiro, Bill. "The Postmodern Guide to Cold Relief." *Health*. Jan.-Feb.1997, 99-102.

Springen, Karen. "Surviving Colds and Flu: Natural Ways to Pamper Yourself During the Sneezing Season." *Vegetarian Times*. December 1993, 82-84.

Springer, Ilene. "Uncommon Remedies for the Common Cold." *Ladies Home Journal*. Dec. 1995, 82-87.

Stapley, Christina. "All You Need is Lovage..." *Herb Quarterly*. Winter 1993, 14-16.

Stoffman, Phyllis. *The Family Guide to Preventing and Treating 100 Infectious Diseases*. New York: John Wiley & Son, 1995.

Tanny, Armand. "Facts to Fight the Common Cold." *Muscle and Fitness.* Jan. 1992, 138-42.

Tarkan, Laurie. "A Guide to the Best Cold Medications." *Good House-keeping.* November 1995, 201-202.

Tenney, Louise. *Today's Herbal Health for Children: A Comprehensive Guide to Understanding Nutrition and Herbal Medicine for Children.* Oak Grove, UT: Woodland Publishing, 1996.

——. *Today's Herbal Health: The Essential Reference Guide to Understanding Herbs Used for Medicinal Purposes.* Pleasant Grove, UT: Woodland Books, 1992.

Tierra, L.. *The Herbs of Life.* Freedom, CA: Crossing Press, 1992.

Tyler, V.E. *Herbs of Choice: The Therapeutic Use of Phytomedicinals.* London: Haworth Press, 1994.

——. *The Honest Herbal* (3rd ed.). New York: Pharmaceutical Products Press, 1993.

Ullman, Dana. *The One Minute Or So Healer.* Los Angeles: Jeremy Tarcher, 1991.

University of Virginia Student Health Website Editors. "Common Non-prescription Cold Medicines." University of Virginia Student Health Website, May 20, 1996.

Vuhovic, Laurel. "99 Home Remedies." *Natural Health.* May/June 1997, 86-96.

——. "Common Colds: 10 Simple Treatments for Congestion, Sore Throat and Fever." *Natural Health.* Jan.-Feb. 1993, 96-98.

——. "Home Remedies: Natural Solutions for Everyday Ailments." *Natural Health.* Sept.-Oct. 1997, 142-145.

Wade, Carlson. *The Home Encyclopedia of Symptoms, Ailments and Their Natural Remedies.* West Nyack, NY: Parker Publishing Co., 1991.

Werbach, Melvyn. "Colds." In *Healing Through Nutrition.* New York: HarperCollins, 1993.

Weiner, M. and Weiner, J. *Herbs That Heal: Prescription for Herbal Healing.* Mill Valley, CA: Quantum Books, 1994.

Weiner, M. *Weiner's Herbal.* Mill Valley, CA: Quantum Books, 1990.

Weiss, R.F. *Herbal Medicine.* Portland, OR: Medicinnia Biologica, 1983.

Wilen, Joan and Wilen, Lydia. *Chicken Soup and Other Folk Remedies.* New York: Fawcett Columbine, 1984.

Willard, T. *The Wild Rose Scientific Herbal.* Calgary, Alberta: Wild Rose College of Natural Healing, 1991.

Zand, Janet , Walton, Rachel, and Rountree, Bob. *Smart Medicine for a Healthier Child: A Practical A to Z Reference to Natural and Conventional Treatments for Infants and Children.* New York: Avery Publishing, 1994.

Index